EATING AND ALLERGY

**Arthritis, Ulcers, Migraine, Heart Disease, Hyperactivity, Depression . . .
are they caused by what we eat?**

ROBERT EAGLE

THORSONS PUBLISHING GROUP
Wellingborough · New York

First published in Great Britain 1979
This revised and reset edition 1986

British Library Cataloguing in Publication Data

Eagle, Robert
  Eating and allergy: arthritis, ulcers, migraine,
  heart disease, hyperactivity, depression —
  are they caused by what we eat?
  1. Food allergy
  I. Title
  616.97'5   RC596

ISBN 0-7225-1279-1

Printed and bound in Great Britain

EATING AND ALLERGY

An invaluable book highlighting the health problems that can result from the food we eat, and investigating the wide gulf between health care and our growing knowledge of allergies.

Contents

		Page
	Foreword	7
Chapter		
1.	Allergies Diagnosed	9
2.	The Medical Controversy	26
3.	Environments: The One We Inhabit and the One We Inherit	55
4.	Diagnosis and Desensitization	75
5.	Drugs for Allergy	108
6.	The Little Children Suffer	114
7.	Coeliac Disease — Inherited or Ingested?	122
8.	Hyperactive Children	126
9.	Migraine and Mental Disorders	132
10.	Obesity and Alcoholism	146
11.	Arthritis	155
12.	Healthy and Not So Healthy Food	162
	Appendix I: Immunological Classification of Allergies	173
	Appendix II: A Review of Methods for Diagnosing and Treating Food Allergy	177
	Appendix III: Food Families	179
	Appendix IV: Hidden Foods	180
	Appendix V: Additives	182
	References and Further Reading	188
	Index	190

I am grateful to the many professional specialists who have helped me with background information for this book and who have provided me with case histories. Although the cases cited are all genuine, the names of patients have been changed for the sake of confidentiality, and any similarity between the names of patients in the book and those of persons living or dead is purely coincidental.

Foreword

It is not a bad thing that the medical profession is slow to adopt new ideas. Patients expect doctors to be cautious and it has been said that there are three stages in the adoption of a new idea in medicine: first, it is dismissed by most doctors as ridiculous. Next, they say: 'it is possible, but where is the proof? Finally, they all find it obvious and claim that they knew it all along.

As Robert Eagle explains so clearly in this new edition of his book *Eating and Allergy*, the evidence that food allergy can give rise to all manner of symptoms is now overwhelming and requires to be taken into consideration in the diagnosis of every case in which the symptoms have no obvious cause.

Allergy to specific foods and chemicals has become a major factor in the physical and mental illnesses peculiar to twentieth-century civilization and needs to be understood not only by doctors but by everybody living in a developed country today.

In fact, already, the whole spectrum of food and chemical allergy including symptoms, diagnosis, treatment and research is covered by a new medical speciality known as clinical ecology, the practice of which is taught and studied at conferences and seminars all over the world.

In the USA where the subject was first developed, the American Academy of Environmental Medicine has been set up to promote what they call 'The Discipline of Clinical Ecology'. Similar medical societies are active in Australia and the United Kingdom, growing in influence and attracting doctors from other countries to their meetings.

With his background in medical journalism and contacts with the leading authorities in clinical ecology, Robert Eagle is well qualified to write a book for the non-medical reader on what this new branch of medicine is all about.

As a doctor and psychiatrist who has been using the ecological approach for many years, I can recommend his book to anyone who suspects that their health is being affected by allergy to one or more of the thousands of new chemicals and food combinations encountered in our increasingly artificial modern environment.

RICHARD MACKARNESS MB, BS, DPM (London)
Consultant Psychiatrist
Alcohol, Drug & Forensic Branch
Mental Health Division
Health Commission of Victoria

Author of:
Eat Fat & Grow Slim, Harvill (1958), Fontana (1961) revised 1975
Not All in the Mind, Pan (1976)
Chemical Victims, Pan (1980)
A Little of What You Fancy, Fontana (1985)

1
Allergies Diagnosed

Barely two weeks before the world's top golfers were to gather in Chicago for the prestigious Western Open golf tournament, a Chicago doctor received an anguished telephone call from the wife of one of the principal contenders.

'Ted, you've got to help,' the voice begged. 'Billy has been acting up for days. He has been following that diet you recommended, but he is still as sassy and irritable as ever. He can't concentrate on his practice and he keeps worrying that he is going to make a mess of the Western Open.'

Mrs Casper was certain that her husband was not just suffering from pre-match nerves — that was not like him. But what she did have good reason to suspect was that Billy's condition was due to something in his diet.

Not many months previously Billy Casper had had to give up playing in almost all the professional golf tournaments in the southern states. At first he had been at a loss to explain why his skill invariably went to pot in the South. As an inhabitant of Salt Lake City he was well enough accustomed to hot weather, so he hardly felt inclined to blame the temperature. And he was puzzled by the fact that his attacks of irritability only came on at certain courses. He could play happily and confidently on all courses in the northern states and on one or two in the South, but simply stepping out onto the green in most southern courses gave him a headache and made him feel miserable.

Seasoned professional golfers are as much prey to the vicissitudes of emotion as the rest of humanity, and yet the circumstances convinced Billy Casper that his problems were not all in his head. But it took some months of discussing the matter with colleagues, friends and doctors before he stumbled across the explanation.

He found that all the golf courses which brought on his symptoms were regularly sprayed with pesticides.

At that time one of the few American doctors interested in the effects of atmospheric pollution on people was Doctor Ted Randolph of Chicago. True, there were a number of specialists — toxicologists — whose job it was to study the possible hazards of man-made chemicals in the environment, but their influence on government policy and public opinion was still slight. Ted Randolph had come to the conclusion that atmospheric pollution was a major threat to health in the early 1950s after successfully diagnosing and treating patients with a variety of ills that could only be attributed to exposure to chemicals which most people appeared to suffer quite happily.

In fact Dr Randolph's preoccupation in those years had been as much with food as with pollutants. He was convinced that many diseases were casued by patients' allergies to particular foods in their diet and that, more often than not, the foods which caused them problems were among those they ate most frequently. It was natural, therefore, that when Billy Casper came to consult Dr Randolph about his apparent reaction to pesticides, the doctor should have put him through a series of tests to see whether he was allergic to any foods as well.

When Mrs Casper called Dr Randolph the investigation of Billy's food allergies was still in its quite early stages. By eliminating foods which he commonly ate from his diet and observing how he fared, they had already concluded that beef and lamb were not doing him any good, and Mrs Casper had ensured that they were taken out of his diet. As a substitute she had been cooking him chicken.

In Dr Randolph's experience patients who had sensitivities or allergies generally reacted to more than one food or chemical. He was therefore not particularly surprised to find that Billy Casper got his symptoms after eating commercially-raised beef as well as inhaling minute quantities of pesticide. Although very few of his medical colleagues shared his beliefs, Randolph's approach appeared to have helped several hundred of his patients. His theories were highly controversial, but as far as he was concerned, his technique was highly effective and based on many years' personal clinical experience.

And it was experience rather than any detailed diagnostic test which made Randolph suggest to Mrs Casper that she should stop feeding her husband chicken. 'It's a hundred to one he is allergic to chicken too,' he told her. 'Take him off the chicken for the next ten days and I'll bet he will win the Western Open hands down. And to put it to the test the evening after the match is over my wife and I will treat you and Billy to a chicken dinner — and see what happens.'

Mrs Casper did as she was advised and Billy did indeed win the Western Open. That evening he and his wife were banqueted in the Randolph home, and the main course was chicken. The next morning the formerly triumphant Casper was as lugubrious and irritable as he had been two week earlier. Being a strict Mormon he had taken no alcohol with the meal but was suffering from all the symptoms of a heavy hangover. It was indeed a hangover, Dr Randolph declared — a chicken hangover!

This anecdote is hardly likely in itself to convince orthodox medical opinion of the reality of food and chemical allergy. In fact in many ways it includes all the ingredients that tend to provoke the conventional mistrust of this controversial subject. Firstly, for instance, Billy Casper's symptoms were mental rather than physical and could not therefore be measured or assessed by an 'objective' observer. Many of the illnesses which food allergists say they can cure are psychological, and this tends to make physically orientated doctors mistrustful. Then again they might ask how a common food such as chicken can give one patient symptoms but leave the majority of us unaffected. Although it is undeniable that some people are very allergic to certain foods and react to them violently and quickly with a swollen mouth, breathing problems or acute stomach upset, this is obviously not the same type of problems our golfing champion suffered.

Nevertheless there is now a great deal of evidence to suggest that allergies to common foods and chemicals are causing a vast mount of sickness which is misunderstood and improperly treated by most doctors. The causes of these allergies are largely unknown, and this book will go into what is and what is not known about them. One belief is that allergies to foods are sparked off by our bodies' reactions to the chemicals which now pervade our air, water, food and medicines. Smoking and the contraceptive pill have been blamed for causing food allergies in otherwise healthy people. Here is another case history. It is not presented as proof of the link between chemicals and food allergy — which we shall investigate later on — but as an everyday example.

Catharine, who is now twenty-five years old and married, had always enjoyed good health as a child and teenager. When she was nineteen she started smoking, and a year later she went on the Pill. The first contraceptive pill she was prescribed made her put on weight, so she was put on to another, milder one which seemed to suit her very well. Two years later, however, she began to get flushes accompanied by a racing pulse. She could not think of any cause for this, until one day when she was on holiday she spoiled herself by eating half a packet of biscuits. Barely fifteen minutes later her face had turned bright red, the veins in her arms and temple were standing out, her pulse had shot up to an alarming rate, and shortly afterwards she was violently sick. She subsequently realized that her symptoms had appeared whenever she had eaten foods like bread or biscuits which contain a lot of wheat flour.

About a year after Catharine's episode with the biscuits a specialist at a leading London hospital came out with the warning that women who were on the Pill and who smoked were very prone to food allergies which could cause a wide variety of symptoms (see page 133). About three quarters of all the women on the Pill who attended her migraine clinic had been found to be allergic to wheat. Many got better when they gave up oral contraceptives, and nearly all of them got better when they avoided foods containing wheat. Catharine decided that she did not want to give up the Pill, but she did find that by avoiding wheat she suffered no more of her attacks. On the few occasions when she has since tested herself on bread or biscuits she has invariably had flushes, racing pulse and acute nausea. Medical tests have shown that she does not have coeliac disease, an illness which is brought on by intolerance of wheat protein. Sometimes, though, she still gets mild attacks of her symptoms after eating sauces or batter which contain small amounts of wheat flour.

Ever since the term 'allergy' was invented in 1906 it has been the subject of controversy — or, to be more accurate, it has been the subject of controversy among doctors. It has been known for centuries that some people react badly to dust, fluff from hairy animals like cats and horses, and foods. It was the Latin poet Lucretius writing in the first century BC who coined the saying 'One man's meat is another man's poison.' And centuries before him, the Greek physician Hippocrates warned that particular foods or changes in diet made some unfortunate individuals ill. For most of us allergy is simply a matter of not being able to tolerate something, be it a food, pollen, chemical or perhaps even a person. Among doctors, however, scientific definitions of allergy have been the subject of hot debate.

The word 'allergy' was first used by an Austrian doctor, Clemens von Pirquet. He was one of the pioneers of immunization, and in the course of his work he found that certain people became hypersensitive to micro-organisms injected into their skin. Normally when a person was given an injection of a diphtheria germ he or she would subsequently develop an immunity to the disease. A minority, however, reacted very badly to the introduction of these foreign cells and would develop widespread rashes or sometimes even suffer an anaphylaxis, a condition in which you choke and go into shock.

Immunity and allergy, von Pirquet suggested, were like opposite sides of the same coin. In most people the body's immune system, or defence forces, was able to overcome the invading bug, and by so doing learned how to deal with it whenever it tried to invade the body again. In allergic people the defence forces overreacted and waged full-scale war on the invader rather than routing it in a little skirmish. The immune system reacts to all foreign matter which enters the body and is usually able to tell the difference between harmless and dangerous substances. But in the allergic person it appears to make an error of judgement and gets terribly steamed up about something most bodies would deal with with minimum fuss.

Von Pirquet's observations about allergy being a state of 'altered reactivity' were made when the subject of immunology was in its infancy. Soon the idea of 'antigens' and 'antibodies' was introduced: antigens are foreign proteins and antibodies are substances produced in the blood to deal with them. What happens in allergy is that many more antibodies are produced than are necessary to cope with the invading antigens, and these spare antibodies go rampaging around causing inflammation. (More detailed explanations of the immune system appear in the next chapter and in Appendix I.)

At first the antigen /antibody idea was regarded with some scepticism by most doctors. It was based on circumstantial evidence and no one had finally proved that antibodies even really existed; indeed it was only about fifteen years ago that scientists using advanced microscopic techniques were able to show us antibodies. Nevertheless the idea did gain ground over the years, so much so that allergy came to be seen in orthodox medical circles purely and simply as an abnormal antigen /antibody reaction. The old idea of allergy being an inability to tolerate something was redefined by immunologists who were reluctant to explain it in anything but their own modern terms.

It is this narrow definition of allergy which has caused confusion and dissent among doctors and which has led to many patients having their diseases misdiagnosed or neglected. The immunological explanation may account for some of the best-known allergic diseases like asthma, eczema, hay fever and the colic suffered by babies who are weaned on cow's milk. But according to a growing body of medical opinion, it does not account for a very wide range of other complaints, both physical and mental, which are brought on by foods and chemicals. These doctors believe that arthritis, depression, schizophrenia, alcoholism, obesity, stomach ulcers, bed-wetting, possibly many cancers, and a host of other plagues are the result of an individual person's intolerance of common foods and/or environmental pollution. Because these doctors have not been able to show that all these diseases are caused by an abnormal immunological reaction, their claims have been dismissed by the medical establishment. Nevertheless there is now a great deal of evidence to suggest that they are right and that the narrow definition which has been foisted on allergy will have to be extended considerably. It also looks as though a great deal of disease which has either been regarded as incurable or which has been put down to 'psychological' factors can be relieved by simple and generally very safe methods.

We shall go into these theories and the facts behind them later on, but perhaps the best way to introduce them is with some illustrative case histories.

Jim Strong* is a dairyman working on a ranch in Wyoming but a few years ago his employment prospects looked bleak. In his late forties he had developed rheumatoid arthritis, the chronic inflammatory disease which affects the connective tissues around the joints. The pain and inflammation in his knees and feet had turned him into a near cripple. To do his job he had to be reasonably fit, but the way his disease was developing made it look as if he would soon be hobbling off into premature retirement. Over a period of about three years he consulted several doctors, and eventually sought help from the famous Mayo Clinic.

One of the perquisites of Jim's job, and one which he availed himself of liberally, was free milk. For years he had drunk up to a gallon of milk a day. He realized that this was an unusual habit, and had mentioned it to his doctors, but had been told that it had no relevance to his arthritis. He was treated with cortisol, the steroid drug, which brought some relief but did not seem to be checking the inexorable development of his disease.

During this period of treatment he developed another complaint, a stomach ulcer. As is normal practice he was put on a bland diet based largely on milk. His arthritis symptoms promptly got worse: indeed he felt so miserable that he could not eat for almost a week. His symptoms began to relent during this fast, and on the seventh day he decided to try the milky diet again. His first meal was followed by a savage resurgence of pain in his joints, together with headache and stomach ache.

This train of events convinced him that his doctors were wrong when they said that milk was harmless. So he had himself

---

*The cases cited here and elsewhere in the book all come from the records of British and American doctors. For the sale of confidentiality the patients' names have been changed.

discharged from the Mayo Clinic and later consulted a doctor in Colorado not far from his home who specialized in treating food allergies. He arrived at the doctor's office on crutches. After hearing his story the doctor advised him to give up milk altogether. Within a few weeks Jim had replaced his crutches with walking sticks, and after three months he was just using a cane. After six months he had thrown his cane away and was back at work. He has not been troubled by ulcers again.

It would be silly to suggest from this single case that rheumatoid arthritis — a disease which has been occupying the attention of some of the best medical brains for many years — is caused only by milk allergy. For the great majority of people this would be quite untrue; but for Jim at least it did seem to play a crucial role in his illness.

Jane Bruff's complaint was very different. A thirty-seven-year-old married Englishwoman who kept a fruit shop, she had become increasingly concerned about her recurrent bouts of palpitations and shortness of breath. Quite out of the blue she would suffer 'attacks' of very rapid heartbeat, which made her feel alarmed and panicky. She was able to put up with these funny turns at home, but when she began to get them in the street, where she felt vulnerable and visible, she really began to worry. Eventually the fear of having an attack in public forced her to take a taxi even for the two-hundred-yard trip down the street to her fruit shop. If possible she preferred to stay indoors, and she became very anxious at the thought of having to step too far outside the familiar safety of her home.

Jane had not kept her suffering to herself; she had consulted her GP and a heart specialist. At first they had suspected that she might be suffering from the effect of a pulmonary embolism (a small clot of blood in the lung) but a chest X-ray showed that this was not the problem. She was prescribed sotalol, a drug used to ease angina and correct abnormalities of the heart rhythm, but it did her no good. As her mother had died from a heart attack not many years before, Jane was worried that the same fate was about to befall her, and she expressed her fears volubly to her doctors.

Her persistent distress, combined with the fact that she showed no sign of having an identifiable organic problem, only succeeded in getting her labelled as a 'problem patient'. Her specialist eventually told her that she had a 'cardiac neurosis'. He took her off the sotalol and prescribed vitamin B tablets, which were not really expected to make her better but were just given as a kind of token reassurance that something was being done.

Fortunately for Jane, a hospital consultant in her area had recently taken an interest in food allergy and had decided to test whether or not it was a genuine disease. He had spread the word among his colleagues that he was prepared to take on patients who were obviously suffering from something mental or physical which had not yielded to conventional diagnosis. It's not often that doctors get such a chance to rid themselves of 'neurotic' patients, and the consultant's invitation was accepted. Early in 1977 Jane was referred to his clinic.

As the consultant was on the lookout for unusual eating habits, he asked Jane about her diet. She promptly admitted that she was a 'tea fiend,' and that she sometimes drank a dozen or more cups of tea a day. Though tea drinking is a beloved British habit, the consultant wondered whether her consumption of vast quantities of the traditional brew might not be the cause of her problems, and he devised a simple way of putting this to the test.

She was asked to come to the clinic several times. Each time she came, she went through the mild but necessary indignity of having a flexible plastic tube inserted through her nose, down her throat and into her stomach. The doctor then took an opaque syringe filled with either coffee, tea or water, and flushed the contents down the tube. As the syringe was opaque she could not see what was in it, and as the liquid bypassed the taste buds in her tongue and palate she could not tell what it was by taste either. She was then wired up to an electrocardiograph, a machine which records the speed and rhythm of the heart, and she was left sitting in a chair accompanied by a nurse and with the consultant popping in for the occasional friendly word.

The consultant had learned that if a patient could not tolerate a certain food, adverse effects might not appear until some time after the food had been taken, so he was content to wait and let things take their course. Indeed, on the occasions when Jane was fed water through the tube nothing happened at all. When she was given coffee or tea, however, the effect was delayed but very violent. Two hours passed as Jane, the nurse and the doctor waited. After two and a half hours, without any warning, her pulse recorded on the electrocardiograph suddenly shot up from the regular normal 70 beats a minute to 250 beats, a highly abnormal and alarming rate, which brought back her old feeling of panic.

The fact that tea and coffee, but not water, should bring on this symptom was pretty convincing evidence that Jane was sensitive to something in those beverages. To clinch the diagnosis Jane was asked to give them both up altogether. And it worked; within a very short time she had lost all her symptoms, was happy to walk down the street, and had returned to her job and a normal social life.

The common ingredient of tea and coffee is caffeine, a stimulant drug in its own right. Several cups of strong coffee can give many people a rapid pulse, though very few experience Jane's aggravated symptoms. Strangely, Jane and her doctor discovered that tomatoes could bring on her attacks too. Though we do not usually think of tomatoes as drugs, they do in fact contain synephrine, a substance which can similarly increase the heart rate. Jane was obviously many times more sensitive to these stimulants than most of us.

A problem which bedevils any attempt to assess a medical therapy impartially is a phenomenon known as the placebo response. *Placebo* is the Latin for 'I shall please', and it has long been recognized that quite a large proportion of people will respond well to almost any treatment you offer them. In trials of new drugs, for instance, patients are given either the real drug or a 'dummy', a chemically inert placebo pill. Although an effective drug should have greater benefits in the long term than a placebo, in the short term it is often very difficult to be sure whether even a potent proven medicine is really any more effective than the dummy. It has been found that up to 50 per cent of us, even when quite seriously ill, will feel better — often for weeks at a time —

if we are given a placebo while believing that we are receiving a potent drug. The placebo response plays a big part in even the most sophisticated medical and surgical procedures; for instance, heart surgeons in the sixties found that patients who underwent a then fashionable kind of heart operation for angina responded little better than patients with the same disease who just went through a dummy operation. Anaesthetic and a few stitches in the chest was enough to convince them they had been cured!

It is not only the placebo response which makes it difficult to assess the real benefits of treatment. The doctor himself is not an impartial observer; he has a vested interest in curing his patients and is often only too prone to make a more favourable assessment of his patients' condition than an unbiased outsider might.

The reason I mention all this is that in the two cases I have just described there is no final proof that the patients' cure was not a super-placebo response to the attentions of a kindly physician. The circumstancial evidence may be compelling, but when one is assessing the merits of an unusuals or unorthodox therapy, one should insist on exacting standards of objectivity.

In the tests the consultant made on a number of other patients referred to him, he made sure that neither he nor the patient knew what was in the syringe used for 'feeding'. One of these patients was Mary Connor, a young woman in her early thirties, whose relationship with her fiancé was in a state of collapse due to her unusual and extremely embarrassing complaint.

Ever since she had been a girl Mary had suffered from attacks of nausea. Her problem was not just stomach ache; she was subject to violent and uncontrollable fits of vomiting which seized her without warning. When she was not actually vomiting, she felt almost permanently queasy. When she was a teenager she had noticed that her fingers would occasionally swell up and at the same time her eyes would feel sore and gritty.

Mary suspected that her diet might have something to do with her nausea, and when she was in her twenties she had become a vegetarian. But she still suffered. Her doctor prescribed antihistamines to control the vomiting, but they were only partially effective. In fact, as time went by she got worse. She became depressed and lost all her zest. Though her boyfriend was sympathetic, her increasing irritability and her decreasing interest in sex were rapidly wearing him out too. Her crisis came when she vomited over the table at a friend's birthday party, after which she refused to eat in public again.

Her baffled GP grew particularly worried about her condition when she told him that she was having fainting fits too. Concerned that she might be suffering from epilepsy, he referred her to a neurologist, who was unable to find anything wrong with her brain. But as she had mentioned that one of her faints had been preceded by palpitations, and that it occurred just after she had had a cup of tea, she was passed on to Dr Finn, the consultant who had treated Jane Bruff.

Mary went through similar tests. During a series of appointments at the clinic she was fed water or tea through a plastic tube. This time, to ensure that he was not unconsciously giving her a clue to the contents of the syringe, Dr Finn asked his nurse to pass him the syringe without letting him or Mary know what was in it. Five times Mary was given water, five times she received tea. When she had water, nothing happened; each time she was given tea she vomited within half an hour. The odds against such a result happening by chance were a thousand and twenty-four to one.

Again, to clinch the diagnosis, they had to see what would happen if she gave up tea. Five months later the doctor was able to report in the *Lancet* that by avoiding tea Mary had lost all her nausea, had given up all drugs, no longer suffered from car sickness, and enjoyed a happy social life. 'She has recently married and is now pregnant,' he concluded.

In that same report to the *Lancet* Dr Finn detailed another three cases in which tea or coffee were clearly responsible for severe, unpleasant and previously untreatable illnesses.

A twenty-six-year-old married man, who had given up work and had been housebound for several years because he suffered from frequent throbbing headaches, had gone through pretty well every available test for brain abnormalities. He had had a skull X-ray, a brain scan, an EEG (electroencephalogram) test to monitor the electrical activity in his head, and an air encephalogram. He had been prescribed drugs used to treat migraine, and when he later developed shooting pains in his spine and told his doctor that he was regularly being caught short by an urgent need to urinate, his kidneys had been examined by yet another X-ray technique. When all these tests had failed to reveal a cause for his pain, he was referred to a psychiatrist.

His wife was reluctant to believe that he had a mental rather than physical disease, and she called for a second opinion. When the consultant asked him about his eating and drinking habits, he admitted to drinking more than twenty cups of coffee a day. Once he gave up his coffee — which required considerable effort — his symptoms disappeared and he was soon feeling well enough to get back to work.

Like Jane Bruff, forty-four-year-old Alan MacNulty complained of chest pains and feelings of panic so severe that he had been admitted to a hospital with a suspected coronary. But his doctors discharged him a few days later when they had been unable to confirm this diagnosis. As distressed as ever, Alan lost interest in his work and began taking a great deal too much time off from the garage where he worked as manager.

As his doctors had now begun to suspect that his troubles were in the mind, he was referred to a psychologist, who gave him twenty sessions of hypnosis, which did little good. He was then referred to a psychiatrist, who subjected him to thirteen bouts of electroconvulsive therapy (ECT) before deciding that this had not really done him much good either.

By now Alan was really depressed and was contemplating suicide. Fortunately at this stage he was referred to Dr Finn — whose interests were not confined to food allergy — for a second opinion on another of his ailments: high blood pressure. Finn found that there was a stenosis, or narrowing, in an artery leading to one of his kidneys, and after this had been successfully repaired by a surgeon, his blood pressure returned to normal. Unfortunately his depression and lethargy did not disappear, and he was taking quantities of tranquillizers.

Eventually it came out that he too was a keen tea and coffee drinker. Three days after acting on advice to avoid everything containing caffeine he began to feel better. Within a few weeks he was back at work, with his mental illness no more than a memory.

Just to demonstrate how diverse the symptoms of tea sensitivity can be, I should mention the case of twenty-six-year-old Robert Potter, a university student, who had been having such severe abdominal pains for three years that he was thought to be suffering from renal colic. All the tests on his kidneys had shown that this could not be the problem, however.

Robert diagnosed his allergy for himself. He told the consultant that his pains were worse when he had been drinking tea or alcohol, and that when he gave these drinks up his symptoms appeared much less frequently. When he went through the same feeding tests as Dr Finn's other patients, it was found that alcohol and tea gave him a very rapid heartbeat which was always followed the next day by his old colicky pain. Though he liked tea and booze as much as any twenty-year-old student, giving them up was amply rewarded by the disappearance of his pain — for good.

As the cases we have seen so far seem to make tea and coffee look like the principal culprits, here is another extract from our consultant's case book, where the symptoms were quite different and caused by a quite different food.

Sue Clark came to the clinic when she was only thirteen years old. Ever since early childhood she had suffered from painful and disfiguring aphthous ulcers on her mouth and in her vagina. Like the other patients she had tried pretty well every treatment available, several of which had unpleasant side effects, but none of which had done the least good. She had been through a battery of tests, all of which had failed to throw any light on the matter. In fact she had been coming to see the consultant long before he became interested in food allergy. Because she was so young and was beginning to spend more time away from school due to her persistent pain and depression about her unpleasant illness. she was one of his most distressing cases.

Dr Finn put her on a meat and water diet for a few weeks, eliminating all cereals, fruit and vegetables. After Sue had been on this meat-only diet for three weeks she was looking a lot better. Not only did she cheer up, but she had only got one more small ulcer. The old ulcers, which had once been the size of a 1p coin, were healing up. Gradually the various foods which she used to eat were reintroduced to her diet one by one, and she and her mother were asked to look out for any reactions which occurred in the following days. It soon became obvious that potato, coffee and chocolate were doing her no good; within a day or two after taking any one of them she would develop fresh ulcers. It was potato that seemed to produce the worst reactions, and at this stage of the proceedings Sue's mother mentioned to the doctor that she cooked chips for the family twice a week. When Sue had been a little girl she had got into the habit of eating pieces of the raw potato while her mother was cooking. She had developed such a liking for raw potato that she began to visit her grandmother in the flat upstairs whenever she was cooking chips, and would help herself to a handful of the raw potato slices. So for many years she had been eating raw potato almost every day. When Sue stoppped eating potato her ulcers stopped troubling her.

Of course most of us can eat potato, raw or otherwise, without getting ulcers. If we could simply say, 'Potatoes cause ulcers', we would expect to see the greater part of the population running around with nasty sores on their faces. What Sue's case and all the other cases I have described suggest is that certain people have an uncommon intolerance to a food and we almost invariably find that this food is a favourite item of the patient's diet and usually the very last thing they would suspect of making them ill.

'Hard cases make bad law' is a legal cliché. It means that court judgements based on highly complicated and individual matters will cause injustice or error if they are applied too widely. The 'hard cases' argument is often heard in medical circles too. There is no shortage of patients with intractable complaints, the origins of which are difficult to diagnose. I am not just talking about diseases like cancer and arthritis, whose causes are obscure, but a whole host of syndromes which seem to be quite peculiar to the individual patient. These syndromes include headaches, palpitations and pains in various parts of the body for which there is no apparent organic cause, as well as psychological symptoms like depression, lethargy and anxiety. It is often hard to pin these symptoms to any well-defined disease, and doctors tend to resort to calling them 'idiopathic' or 'functional'.

An idiopathic or functional complaint is as distressing for the sufferer as any disease with an established diagnostic label, but because its cause is uncertain it tends to arouse alarm and suspicion on the part of the doctor. All of us are inclined to flounder if we are faced with a problem we are supposed to overcome but cannot understand, and doctors probably find themselves in this position more often than most. A patient who is suffering from an undiagnosable condition which does not appear to warrant urgent medical or surgical intervention may be told that the complaint is psychosomatic. This is sometimes a quite fair description, implying rightly enough that mental upsets can cause physical distress, but the patient frequently thinks that the doctor is saying that the symptoms are imaginary or 'all in the mind'.

One of the great problems faced by food allergists is that they have succeeded with patients whose complaints other doctors had previously labelled as psychosomatic. Although you might expect a doctor to be congratulated by his colleagues for solving a 'hard case', the reaction is often quite the reverse. For just as a doctor — prey, like all of us to emotion — is annoyed by his own inability to pin down the causes of idiopathic pains, headaches or anxieties, his pride is doubly affronted when another doctor claims to have cured the patient by applying theories and methods which are controversial or unfamiliar.

When a British doctor, Richard Mackarness, wrote a book (see References, page 188) about food allergies in 1976, he aroused antagonism from the vast majority of his colleagues. By applying a simple but almost unheard-of technique he had helped a patient with severe psychiatric illness who had not been relieved by previous specialist care. This case formed the backbone of his book, and although it aroused a great deal of public interest, the reaction of Dr Mackarness's medical colleagues was that he was trying to make new laws from hard cases. So intense was the feeling against him and his unorthodox methods that he was ostracized by many of his medical colleagues.

Recently, though, atttitudes have begun to change. Shortly after I had written an article in the medical magazine *British Medicine*, in January 1979, on the success American food allergists were enjoying, Dr Mackarness wrote a letter to the editor of that magazine reporting that, 'Some of my hospital colleagues who used to turn and walk the other way when they saw me coming, now actually speak to me. One chap who had been particularly hostile when my book came out, put his arm round my shoulders and said: "You know, Mac, we always thought there was something in what you were doing".'

A revolution indeed. But what has prompted this change in attitude?

2

The Medical Controversy

Summer was not a pleasant season for Dr Charles Blackley. Ever since he was a boy the sunny June days with their light wafting breezes had brought him nothing but misery. Sometimes he wished it would just rain right through until August. Dr Blackley suffered from hay fever.

We now know that hay fever is an allergy to pollen or spores and that if you suffer from it you can often predict to within a few days when you will get your next annual bout of sore eyes, runny nose or asthma. But in the 1870s, when Dr Blackley was practising as a physician in Manchester, no one knew what caused hay fever.

The fact that his main symptoms were a runny nose and sore eyes made him wonder whether the cause might not be something blowing in the wind. The further fact that he suffered his symptoms in the early summer when the trees, grasses and flowers were all blooming made him suspect that pollen was the culprit. So to put his theory to the test he collected samples of pollen by covering glass slides with a sticky substance and exposing them to the air in his garden. He found that his symptoms were almost invariably worse on the days when the slides attracted most pollen. For more conclusive evidence he bravely went out among the flowers and trees and collected more pollen, which he stored in little glass phials until winter, when the plants were no longer in bloom. When he opened the phials and sniffed the pollen he came down with a severe headache, sneezing and all the symptoms of a nasty attack of flu. The reaction was so unpleasant that he never felt tempted to try it again.

His suspicions had proved to be accurate. But he was still left with a question which has puzzled allergists ever since: why doesn't everybody suffer like this?

He was only able to go a little way towards answering that question. He noticed that if a tiny amount of pollen was scratched into his skin, a red mark, or weal, would appear shortly afterwards. He tried this on a number of his patients and found that those who suffered from hay fever got a similar weal, whereas non-sufferers did not. This basic test was the forerunner of one of the diagnostic methods used by allergists today when they are trying to work out which substances their patients are allergic to.

In 1911 two doctors working at St Mary's Hospital in London, Dr L. Noon and Dr J. Freeman, discovered that many patients with pollen allergy could be temporarily cured by giving them a series of injections of the pollen which caused their symptoms. The technique was inspired by the success of immunization techniques against diseases such as smallpox. Starting with extremely small quantities of pollen in special solution they would give their patients increasing doses over a period of several weeks, and at the end of this ordeal — and for many patients it was not a particularly pleasant therapy — they would find that they could tolerate quantities of pollen which would previously have made them very sick.

Although in the early years of this century the diagnosis and treatment of pollen and spore allergies occupied (and still does occupy) the minds of researchers, food allergy was not being neglected. In 1921 Dr Carl Prausnitz and Dr Heinz Küstner conducted a classic experiment which gave an important insight into the mechanism of allergy.

Like most doctors who have ever interested themselves in allergies, they were themselves allergic: Prausnitz to grass pollen and his boss Küstner to fish. Both their allergies were of the acute kind which produces immediate reactions. Prausnitz would suffer from asthma as soon as pollen touched his airways, and whenever Küstner put fish to his lips, his mouth would swell. In their experiment each took a sample of his own blood serum and injected it into his colleague's skin. When a tiny amount of pollen was then injected into Küstner's skin, a large weal immediately appeared on the site. When Prausnitz was challenged with fish, the reaction was similar.

What the experiment showed was that sensitivity to a particular substance could be transferred from one person to another via blood serum. It seemed, therefore, that a vital part of whatever caused allergic reactions was to be found circulating in the blood-stream. It was not long after these doctors had published their findings that a great divide began to open between two schools of medical thought on the subject of allergy. On the one hand there were the immunologists, who were becoming increasingly convinced that the answer to allergy was to be found by closer study of the way the body's defence system worked or failed. This path was to take them ever deeper into the complexities of blood cells and antibodies and their functions and interactions. On the other hand there were the ecologists, who were less interested in the apparently insoluble problems of the immune system, but much more concerned about the wide range of diseases which seemed to result from an individual person's inability to tolerate particular foods or chemicals present in the environment. Leaving the ecologists aside for the moment, let us consider what modern immunology has to say about allergy.

The Immunological Approach

Although it was not until the early 1960s that researchers actually isolated antibodies and were able to examine their chemical structure, the belief that allergy was the result of an abnormality of the immune system attracted increasing numbers of medical men and is now the orthodox approach to allergic diseases. It is probably true to say that immunology gained momentum more quickly in the United States than in Britain. For many years the great majority of British physicians were reluctant to believe that asthma, for instance, could be explained in immunological terms; they tended to explain it away as a psychosomatic disease. This former difference between American and British attitudes is still reflected in the number of doctors in each country who are specialists in allergy. In the United States there are several thousand doctors who can style themselves 'allergists', having passed the exams set by the Board of Allergy and Immunology. In Britain there are relatively few doctors who specialize in allergy full time and there is little scope for young doctors who seek advanced training in the field. American interest in immunology was doubtless fired by the influx into the United States of Jewish doctors from Austria and Germany who had set the pace in immunological research but fled Nazi persecution during the Hitler era. More recently, immunology has been advancing in Britain, but research has concentrated heavily on cancer and diseases such as rheumatoid arthritis.

The basis of immunology is the reaction between antigens (foreign proteins entering the body) and antibodies. Proteins are chains of amino acid molecules consisting of combinations of carbon, hydrogen, oxygen, nitrogen and sometimes sulphur too, and they are an essential ingredient of all organic (living) matter. Any protein can serve as an antigen: viruses, bacteria, food and pollen are just some of the best-known antigen vehicles.

Antibodies are another class of protein, produced by cells in the spleen and lymph glands. When these cells, which are in fact white blood cells called B-lymphocytes, come across an antigen they undergo a transformation and release antibody. The function of antibody is to combine with the antigen and thus render it harmless. Even in a healthy person it can take some days for enough antibody to be produced to knock out the antigen. But once this has happened, you have a long lasting protection (immunity) from the antigen. This explains why most people only suffer from infectious diseases like measles and chicken pox once in their life; when the virus enters the body a second time there are already immunological resources at hand to get rid of it quickly. This is also the principle behind vaccination: you are injected with a small amount of antigen which is not enough to give you raging symptoms but which is enough to alert the white cells to produce antibody to deal with any future attack.

An important characteristic of antibodies is that they are highly specialized. An antibody to one antigen offers no protection against any other antigen. The reason why we can suffer from flu every year is that the flu virus — unlike measles or chicken pox — is constantly changing and evolving. The flu virus which makes us ill this year will have undergone a significant metamorphosis by next year, so this year's antibodies will only offer limited immunity.

Immunization against some diseases, notably tetanus, diphtheria and hepatitis, consists of injecting a person with antibodies. This method does not give long-lasting protection, because the body has not learned how to produce antibodies of its own accord. It is therefore used to give short-term protection or to help a patient overcome an actual attack of the disease. If you need long-term protection you have to have regular booster shots. The protection given by an antibody injection is called 'passive immunity'. Longer-lasting protection can be given by injections of the disease virus itself, usually dead or weakened, which prompts your body to make its own antibodies. This usually works well — except in the case of flu just mentioned.

There are in fact four main classes of antibody and each may behave in a variety of ways. The workings of the immune system have already filled many weighty scientific tomes and even so, what we still do *not* know about it is infinitely vaster than what we do know. Very briefly though, we know that some antibodies circulate in the blood while others attach themselves to cells in the tissues of the body. Some antibodies attach themselves to one or other of the various kinds of white blood cells. And as well as antibodies there are white cells which are drawn to foreign proteins or invading organisms and can destroy them without the intervention of antibody.

This is just an outline of the normal immune response. In an allergic person the system malfunctions. Though the symptoms are often obvious and though the immediate cause of some of those symptoms is quite well known, the deep underlying causes are still a mystery. Some allergic people appear to have a lack of a certain kind of white blood cell, and allergies also tend to run in families. But the genetic factor is complicated and unpredictable. For example, one of the most eminent British allergists, Dr Bill Frankland, who suffers from hay fever, has an identical twin brother who has never had an allergy in his life.

Immunologists have classified allergies into four types (see Appendix I). Type One allergy is probably the best known and best understood. It is the kind of complaint suffered by someone who gets an immediate and sometimes almost fatal attack the moment they are exposed to even a minute quantity of the guilty allergen (an allergen being an antigen which arouses an allergy). If you are sensitive to pollen, a few grains of the dust can cause itchy eyes, runny nose or asthma. If you are sensitive to a food, a touch of it on your lips will make them swell; if you are unlucky enough to swallow a piece, your throat may swell and choke you; if the allergen gets as far as your stomach, you will vomit, and if it reaches as far as the intestine, you will get diarrhoea. Admittedly the symptoms are not always quite as violent as this, but you are certainly left in no doubt as to the cause of the problem.

The reason for these sudden reactions is that a group of cells called 'mast cells' have become sensitized to the allergen.

The first time an allergic patient is exposed to the allergen which causes his symptoms he notices nothing at all. But what has happened is that he has produced an abnormal amount of antibody — of a type called Immunoglobulin E, or IgE for short — to the antigen. This IgE then proceeds to get stuck to the mast cells, which are generally situated in the region of the body where the exposure first occurred. One of the properties of mast cells is that they contain large quantities of histamine, bradykinin and a number of other natural chemicals, including one with the most ominous name of 'slow-reacting substance'. The functions of these chemicals are to increase the flow of fluids in and out of blood vessels, to influence the amount and type of fluid produced by mucous glands and to make muscles in internal organs contract. In the normal course of events these substances are being released all the time to regulate our natural functions. But in an allergic person whose mast cells have been covered by IgE, the arrival of a second dose of the allergen puts the cells into frenzied activity. They literally explode, releasing their load of histamine and other chemicals. The result of this onslaught depends upon where the sensitized cells are located. In the nose they will cause a discharge of watery mucus; around the eyes they will cause inflammation and watering; in the bronchial passage they will cause the muscles to contract and make you wheeze; in the gut they will cause diarrhoea. If large enough quantities of the slow-reacting substance are released the result can be catastrophic anaphylaxis in which the airways become closed and blood-pressure drops. This reaction is fortunately not common, but patients who do get it need oxygen and a shot of adrenalin to revive.

The foods which most commonly cause this kind of reaction are fish, shellfish, nuts, eggs and milk. If like the first three items they are easily identifiable, sufferers often don't bother to consult a doctor about the allergy. The allergen is obvious and the way to avoid the reaction is to avoid the food. Nevertheless fish-sensitive people sometimes have an attack simply by walking past a fish market, and an acutely egg-sensitive person may sneeze if someone cracks an egg when he happens to be standing in the kitchen. Egg and milk are very difficult to avoid as they crop up in a vast number of prepared foods. Though there are some medical treatments (which I shall describe later) for this condition , the best cause is to follow a careful diet — admittedly no easy task.

By now you may have realized that the immunologists' ideas about allergies are pretty complicated. The kind of antibody reaction I have just described is only one of four types of reaction which are believed to occur. So that we do not get bogged down in detail at this early stage I have outlined these other types in Appendix I at the back of the book.

The main point to make about the immunological approach to allergy is that it has led researchers deeper and deeper into the intricacies of the immune system. Though they have identified several kinds of antibodies and studies and chemical activity of various types of cell, they have not really come much nearer to finding a cure or a complete explanation for these strange reactions to foods, pollens and chemicals.

But while the immunologists have been focusing on ever smaller aspects of disease, that other group of doctors interested in allergy, the ecologists, have been looking outward and suggesting that the causes and the cures of many diseases can be found there.

The Ecological Approach

Basically the ecologists are less interested in how allergies occur than in what makes them occur. Their observations have convinced them that the answer to disease is to be found in the air we breathe and the food we eat rather than in messing around with blood cells. This is admittedly a sweeping generalization, but it points out the difference between the two schools of thought.

Perhaps the first doctor to practise ecological medicine was a British psychiatrist, Francis Hare. In 1906 he published a vast book — a thousand pages long and in two volumes — called *The Food*

Factor in Disease, in which he declared that migraine, bronchitis, asthma, eczema, gastrointestinal disturbances, epilepsy, angina, high blood-pressure, gout, arthritis and a number of other degenerative diseases were caused by the patient eating more starchy and sugary foods than his body was able to cope with. His evidence for this was that many of his patients had improved dramatically when these carbohydrates were reduced or removed from their diet and replaced with foods rich in protein. If the patient started eating sugary, starchy foods again, his troubles would return.

Despite the great effort Dr Hare had evidently put into writing these two tomes, his ideas were not taken very seriously by his colleagues. His professional status — he was practising in Brisbane, Australia, rather than at a London teaching hospital — probably did not assist his credibility in a conservative profession, and his book was panned in a review in the *Lancet*.

Although not even ecologist doctors would take Hare's every word as gospel today, the idea that disease was caused by food was revolutionary. Remember that we are not talking about food poisoning caused by dirt and contamination, but about the result of an excess of a common food which certain individuals are ill equipped to deal with.

Hare also believed that people who could not handle carbohydrates actually became addicted to them. This may sound paradoxical, but Hare observed that people whose diets consisted largely of sugary, starchy foods would experience withdrawal symptoms of intense irritability and malaise if they stopped eating these foods for a short while. If they persevered and kept carbohydrates out of their diet for several days, these withdrawal symptoms would eventually disappear. Unfortunately what usually happened was that the food-addicted person would rush off to the larder and stuff himself with more carbohydrates as soon as he felt withdrawal symptoms coming on. He would thus become dependent on the foods which were the source of his suffering — a state of affairs which in the long term led to chronic disease. Hare explained alcoholism as an addiction to carbohydrates, and this belief is still upheld by some ecologists.

Medicine is a conservative profession and Dr Hare's ideas were published before their time. But it was not long before other doctors began to say how they had cured diseases caused by sensitivity to foods. In 1908 an English doctor, A. T. Schofield, explained to readers of the *Lancet* how he had discovered that a thirteen-year-old boy was allergic to eggs, which gave him acute asthma. Over a period of seven months Dr Schofield deliberately fed the boy minute but gradually increasing amounts of raw eggs. He began with a solution which contained one part in ten thousand of egg, and slowly increased the dose so that by the end of six months the lad had consumed a total of one egg. During the following month the boy managed to eat four whole eggs without getting his asthma.

Four years later a New York doctor, Oscar Schloss, successfully treated an eight-year-old who had a similar allergy. Not content with discovering that eggs were to blame for the boy's misery, Dr Schloss tried to work out which part of the egg was responsible. After a long series of tests he concluded that a particular egg protein, ovomucoid, prompted the most violent reactions. He then treated the boy by giving him three capsules a day containing two milligrams of ovomucoid. He gradually increased the dose, and after ten weeks the boy could eat two eggs at a time without falling ill.

In 1921 Dr William Duke, who practised in Kansas City, published a report in the medical journal *Archives of Internal Medicine* detailing cases which made it plain that eggs, milk and wheat made some people suffer severe stomach upsets. He then went on to produce evidence that food allergies could cause bladder pain and even Ménière's syndrome, a disease of the inner ear which gives you headaches and vertigo. He found he could give his patients an attack of their symptoms by feeding them the food to which they were allergic or by injecting food extracts into their skin. He reported that the reaction to these provocation tests was often so strong that his poor patients needed a shot of adrenalin to bring them back to normal.

After a few more years of treating patients with a wide variety of complaints Dr Duke realized that what he called 'specific hypersensitiveness' to particular foods carried important implications. Here, he wrote, 'we have a subject which deals with illnesses caused by inert matter. It is nevertheless as broad and as important as the illnesses caused by living matter such as bacteria.'

Perhaps the most eminent and methodical pioneer of ecological medicine was Dr Albert Rowe. As a young physician working in Oakland, California, in the 1920s he was eager to keep up with the latest medical research, most of which at that time was being done in Europe. One day he came across a book written in French by two Parisian doctors, Richet and Saint Girons, titled *L'Anaphylaxie Alimentaire*. In this book, which they wrote in 1919, the two Frenchmen had gathered together pretty well all the available accounts of illnesses caused by food. They described for the most part the typical acute reactions in which the allergic patient got swollen lips, itchy, runny nose and eyes, asthma or stomach upset shortly after tasting a particular food. They also mentioned, though they were unable to explain, how delayed reactions like eczema also affected some people who suffered from food allergies.

This book so intrigued Dr Rowe that he persuaded his wife, who spoke French, to help him translate it into English. His interest was not just academic; he wanted to put the Frenchmen's ideas into practice.

Rowe quickly realized that it was going to be no easy task to sort out the problems of people who were allergic to common foods. Patients who got a sharp, almost immediate reaction to something they ate only occasionally — like strawberries or water melon — were obviously not hard to identify. They usually came to him already knowing the cause of their problem, and the best advice he could give them was to avoid the food. But a common food, like eggs or milk or wheat, often only caused reactions that showed up hours or days later and were not as dramatic as the immediate reactions. As these foods are staple ingredients mixed together in cooking, the patient found it hard to identify a particular food which was causing him problems. And of course there was no reason why a patient should not be allergic to more than one common food.

One way of testing for allergy was to give the patient an injection of an extract of the food into the skin and to see if it produced a weal or any other reaction. Dr Rowe found that these tests worked reasonably accurately in young children but were less reliable in adults. Sometimes a skin test would give a 'false positive' result; in other words, the reaction would make it look as if the patient was sensitive to a food when he was not. Sometimes a skin test of a food would produce no reaction, even though this food was later found to be allergenic. As these tests seemed to be so fraught with difficulty he devised a better one — the elimination diet.

As its name implies, an elimination diet is designed to eliminate the allergens from the foods you eat. When Rowe drew up his diets he made it plain to his patients that they were not to touch wheat, milk, eggs, apples, bananas, oranges, celery, cabbage, cauliflower, potato, fish and nuts — in other words, the foods which he thought to be the most frequent allergens. He then gave them a list of foods which they could eat, making sure that it included enough meat, vegetables, cereal, sweeteners and cooking oil to make it tasty and attractive. Table I shows three of his elimination diets, listing foods that his patients were allowed to eat.

Table I Three of Dr Rowe's elimination diets

	Diet 1	Diet 2	Diet 3
Cereal	Rice	Corn, maize, tapioca	Rye and rice
Meat	Lamb	Bacon, chicken	Beef
Vegetables	Lettuce, spinach, carrots	Peas, asparagus, artichokes	String beans, tomatoes, beetroot
Fruits	Lemons, pears, peaches	Pineapples, prunes, apricots	Grapefruit, pears, peaches
Miscellaneous	Sugar, olive oil, gelatin, cane syrup	Sugar, corn oil, corn syrup	Sugar, cottonseed oil, gelatin, maple syrup

If you had a suspected allergy you would be put on one of these diets for between five days and a fortnight. If your symptoms had cleared up after this period it could be assumed that you were not allergic to any of the foods in the diet. But if you had not got any better you would be put on another diet or asked to give up one or two suspect items in your first diet. The first stage of treatment was complete once you had found a simple diet which gave no symptoms. From then on you would add new foods to your diet one by one, eating them in quite large quantities, and waiting for a few days to see if your symptoms returned. If they did not return, you could be reasonably assured that the food was safe and go on to add another food. If they did return, the new food was probably the culprit.

The great virtue of this treatment is its simplicity — as long, that is, as you don't cheat yourself by eating prohibited foods on the side. To make the basic diets more acceptable to his patients, Dr Rowe had to become something of a cookery expert. As his patients could not eat wheat bread, for instance, he had to teach them how to make rice bread, rye bread and corn pone, which is a scone made from maize flour.

Dr Rowe had quite startling success with his elimination diets, which impressed many of his contemporaries in the United States and Britain. In an old medical textbook I came across, dated 1934 and titled *Recent Advances in Allergy*, Rowe's work is mentioned more times than that of any other specialist and the author warmly recommends Rowe's diets for the treatment of migraine, asthma, eczema, hives, chronic catarrh, persistent indigestion and other stomach ailments, gastric and duoenal ulcers and mouth ulcers, period pains and a mental condition called 'allergic toxaemia', which according to the author 'is characterized by fatigue, nervousness, mental confusion and aching of the body'.

Perhaps one of Rowe's greatest feats was his success in treating ulcerative colitis, which is an extremely painful inflammation of the bowel. If it is allowed to progress, this condition can become so intractable that a surgeon has to intervene by performing an ileostomy. In this operation a permanent hole is made in the front of the abdomen, which is connected to the small intestine. The unfortunate patient has to spend the rest of his days with a plastic bag attached to his body over this hole to catch the excrement as it comes out. By using elimination diets Rowe was able to bring about a remission of the disease in ten out of fourteen patients with ulcerative colitis he treated.

He was incidentally not the only doctor to do this: an American contemporary, A. F. R. Andresen, had similar success with similar diets. Both concluded that of all the foods to blame for the disease, milk was the commonest offender. This was a particularly horrifying discovery in view of the fact that the standard treatment for ulcerative colitis was a 'bland' diet, whose principal constituent was milk! So it is very possible that many patients were actually made worse by their well-meaning doctors.

Like most doctors who have the skill to treat diseases which defeat their colleagues, Dr Rowe built up a very prosperous private practice, in Oakland, California. In the early 1960s, when he was already an old man, he told a visiting British doctor, Richard Mackarness (who was later to introduce ecological medicine to England), that he earned $193,000 a year after tax. So even though his ideas were clearly no longer widely discussed in orthodox medical textbooks, there were plenty of patients prepared to pay for his help in hard cash.

Although Rowe did have his own ideas about the physical mechanisms in the body which sparked off symptoms, he preferred to treat patients than to do biochemical research. His successors in the field have tended to adopt the same attitude. 'If the treatment works, let's use it' could be their motto. Nor, until recently, have the ecologists been particularly keen on performing the kind of clinical trials which academically inclined doctors insist on. The aim of clinical trials is to work out how much of the therapy is a 'real' response which has nothing to do with the charisma and persuasiveness of the doctor or the suggestibility of the patient. It is largely for these reasons that the beliefs and practices of the ecologists have not won many converts in the teaching hospitals and research institutes which set the tone of orthodox medicine.

Unfortunately the main characteristic of orthodoxy is inertia. Those with power and influence do not take kindly to having their own cherished concepts of what is what challenged. Indeed, even individuals highly placed in the orthodox hierarchy very often come up against a brick wall if they present new ideas which do not 'fit in'. This was to be the fate of Dr Arthur Coca.

Coca, who was born in 1875, could be regarded as a pillar of the contemporary medical establishment. In the 1930s he was professor at Cornell and a leading light in immunological research: he was the founder of the *Journal of Immunology*. He later took a job with the pharmaceutical company Lederle, as its medical director. One day during this latter stage of his career he happened to notice that his wife was avoiding a number of foods she used to eat quite happily.

'What's the matter with them?' he asked. She admitted, somewhat reluctantly, that they made her pulse accelerate in a disagreeable way. 'I wasn't going to mention it to you because I thought you would think I was being neurotic; she added.

Coca suffered from a number of allergies himself — like others I have mentioned, his interest in the subject originated from personal suffering — and as an immunologist he had made a major contribution to the classification of allergic reactions: so he was not one of those who thought allergies were 'just psychosomatic'. But his wife's story struck him as bizarre — until he exposed himself and other patients to allergens and felt the racing pulse for himself.

He went on to find that as well as the rapid pulse there were other unpleasant reactions to food and chemicals which did not fit in with the orthodox immunological concepts.

Laboratory tests sometimes failed to show signs of a chemical or cellular activity to indicate that the offending substance had attracted the attention of the immune system. He therefore speculated that this sort of allergy must be caused by an abnormality or malfunction in some quite separate part of the human physiology. The racing pulses suggested that the sympathetic nervous system could be involved — and he even went as far as having a sympathectomy (a surgical operation which disconnects sympathetic nerves) to see if he was right. Sadly it seems he was only partly right: at least, he lost his sensitivity to some allergens but not to others!

Although he obviously had not solved the whole problem, he was so taken with this form of allergy which did not fit the immunological rules that he developed his findings and conclusions in a book, to which he gave the forbidding but descriptive title *Familial Non-Reaginic Food Allergy*. By 'non-reaginic' he meant a kind of allergy which was not provoked by demonstrable reactions by the immune system. In the book he recommended that doctors should look for the non-reaginic allergies in their patients by taking their pulse before and after they had been fed a food or exposed to a chemical. A marked acceleration indicated an allergy. His pulse test is still widely used by ecologists, though usually in conjunction with other diagnostic methods (see Chapter 4 and Appendix II).

Despite his high standing in academic and immunological circles Coca's new ideas raised nothing but eyebrows among his former colleagues. He also gained a reputation for eccentricity on account of the great precautions he had begun to take to protect himself against invisible allergens in cooked foods. He would not eat in restaurants, and on one occasion when a medical association had invited him to a dinner as the guest of honour, he refused the meal laid before him and ate nothing but the food he had brought with him in a sandwich box. His mistrust of chemical vapours in the atmosphere was equally violent; a fellow doctor who had arrived at his house holding an evening newspaper was brusquely told not to bring *that thing* through the front door lest it sicken him with its toxic fumes. (He was of course referring to the ink in the newsprint rather than the editorial matter.)

Coca felt bitter that the colleagues whose opinion he had respected should ignore his new theory. In the preface to the second edition of his book he complained of:

> considerable provocation at the hands of many personal acquaintances among experienced allergists and other medical specialists, from whom I could reasonably expect at least an unprejudiced hearing, if not generous co-operation. The attitude of most of these towards the first edition of this monograph has been that of a skepticism so uncompromising that I have not even been invited to demonstrate the new method of examination described therein. It is quite out of the question to attribute this attitude to any personal prejudice; no, the reason for it is that the medical profession is again faced with scientific findings and their consequences that are so far out of line with settled concepts as apparently to represent the impossible.

Despite this antagonism from orthodoxy we should remember that this was the second edition of the book, which was very soon to be followed by a third, and some years later by a simplified version for lay people entitled *The Pulse Test*, which apparently still sells well. In other words, it seems that although he was not convincing the doctors in high places, his idea was very popular with many others. The rift between the immunologists and the ecologists was now opened wide.

A few years before Coca's book was published, Herbert Rinkel, a young doctor from Kansas who had graduated top of his year from Illinois' Northwestern University and was now practising as an allergist in Oklahoma City, terrified his family and friends gathered together at his birthday party by crashing to the floor in a dead faint. Although even six-foot-three former full-backs (as he was) are known to faint occasionally, he had done nothing like this before, and his alarmed colleagues immediately feared he had had a coronary. The truth was that he had just taken a bit of angel food cake.

For many years previously Dr Rinkel had suffered from recurrent fatigues and headaches and a very aggravated and distressing rhinitis. His nose did not just run; day after day it seemed to pour out great streams of mucus. This had been embarrassing enough on the football field: in the doctor's office it was professionally disastrous.

Reading Albert Rowe's books and papers on food allergy, Rinkel had wondered whether his complaint was a food reaction. One thing made him suspect strongly that it was: every week since he had been a student his father back in Kansas had sent him a gross of eggs. Rinkel had decided to study medicine when he was already in his twenties and married with a baby son. They had very little money and the eggs made up their staple diet.

Rowe had warned about common foods and drawn particular attention to the allergenicity of eggs. And here was young Rinkel gobbling them a dozen a day. So he decided to find out if he did have an allergy to them.

Unfortunately he did not embark on a formal elimination diet, but tried to see if he could provoke an immediate reaction by swallowing six raw scrambled eggs at once. Nothing happened, and he assumed that the eggs were innocent after all.

It was only six years and many floods of rhinitis later that he thought of trying to make a more methodical search for a food allergen. He stopped eating eggs, which were still one of his favourite foods, and waited to see what would happen.

After the third and fourth days he did seem to be losing his symptoms; but it was still rather early to be certain whether the improvement was real. The sixth day after the start of his eggless diet was his birthday, and the traditional preparations were made for a party. In her enthusiam Mrs Rinkel forgot that her husband was not supposed to be eating eggs, and cracked three big ones into the cake mixture. When the misbegotten confection, decked with candles, was subsequently brought into the party, cut, and a piece offered to the birthday man himself, he was so much into the swing of things that he too forgot about hidden eggs. Ten minutes later he was lying on the floor.

Dr Rinkel did recover from his swoon and naturally began thinking what had caused it. He reasoned that he must have been allergic to eggs, and that his brief abstinence had somehow rendered him even more susceptible than before. But this was almost unbelievable; for years he had eaten eggs ad infinitum; could it be true that barely six days after giving them up, a few egg-laden cake crumbs had all but killed him? The only way to settle his doubts was to go through the whole routine again and see if he got the same reaction. He did.

Now, one of the features of Dr Rinkel's clinic in Oklahoma City was the everlasting parade of patients with intractable ailments — asthma, migraine, palpitations, as well as the rhinitis and general malaise which he had suffered. When Dr Rinkel asked them whether any particular food disagreed with them, they would almost invariably say no. But his own recent experiences made him think that perhaps they were allergic to foods but did not recognize the allergy because they were taking the guilty food regularly every day. After all, he had loved his eggs before trying to do without them.

He duly advised patients to give up one particular item in their diet which they ate a lot of, and a few days later he would stand by them as they took it again for the first time. If they were allergic to it, they would get a rapid attack of their symptoms, not usually a dramatic as his own seizure but acute nevertheless.

He coined the phrase 'masked allergy' for this condition. This concept was rather like Francis Hare's idea of carbohydrate addiction in which the addict was caught in a vicious circle: the more he ate of the food the sicker he became — but he did not recognize the connection because he enjoyed the food so much. The only way out was to give it up. Rinkel could not imagine why re-exposure to the food should provoke an acute reaction, but it seemed to be an effective test for food allergy.

The medical establishment greeted his reports with even less enthusiam than they had accorded Arthur Coca's pulse test. The editor of the *Journal of Allergy* turned Rinkel's paper down flat, thus depriving him of an audience among his colleagues.

This rejection, with its unspoken implication that the editor regarded his observations as unsound, stung Rinkel to the quick. But rather than plead his case with other journals, he decided to pursue his research until he had a mass of data which the most stolid editor could not afford to ignore. Some eight years later, in 1944, his findings were published.

In that same year Rinkel was to meet an ambitious young doctor whose single-mindedness was soon to establish him as the leading exponent of ecological medicine in the United States. Dr Theron G. Randolph, known to his friends as Ted, had recently returned to his native Midwest from Boston, where he had been working in the allergy clinic of one of America's most famous hospitals, Massachusetts General. In Boston he had learned to value Rowe's elimination diets, and when he returned to the Midwest in the middle of the Second World War to take up a teaching post at the University of Michigan he was given the university hospital's allergy clinic to run. He met Herbert Rinkel at a medical meeting at which the Oklahoma physician had been given one of his rare opportunities to lecture on masked allergy, and promptly decided to test this idea for himself. He found that his patients responded just as Rinkel said they would. Moreover, the technique helped him too.

When they had met, Rinkel had stressed that corn was a very common allergen, and warned that Rowe's elimination diets did not take this fact into enough account. Now, over the years Ted Randolph had wondered whether the headaches he suffered were the symptom of a food allergy, but although he had tried Rowe's basic elimination diets on himself, he had to admit that he had not yet followed one which was completely corn-free. The great problem with corn is that it is used to make much of the sugar used in the United States and therefore it is often a hidden factor in the diet. When Randolph subsequently put himself on a corn-free diet his headaches disappeared. This personal experience together with the clinical evidence offered by his patients convinced him utterly.

Nevertheless, when he moved later that year to take up private practice and a new part-time academic post at Northwestern University near Chicago, he found that local professional interest in food allergy was practically nil. So he set about trying to raise some interest.

He began by asking nursing students to help him in a research project. He selected those of obviously robust physique and took details of their eating habits and any illnesses they suffered, and got them to try simple elimination diets and feeding tests. He came to the conclusion that two thirds of them had an obvious history of food allergy. Some reacted to foods they ate infrequently, but most to common foods. At the time many members of the hospital nursing staff and students had been suffering from symptoms of flu and it was thought that the fatigue from working long hours was making them prone to infections. But Ted Randolph boldly suggested that food allergies were to blame.

Around this time he also began to tell colleagues that he thought food allergy was involved in alcoholism, mental disease and many of the chronic aches and pains some patients complain of, but which seem to have no obvious organic origin. His more conservative superiors at Northwestern University thought this was taking things too far. Many did not care for the way he was preaching his controversial ideas to students and nurses, and suspected that he was indulging in gimmickry to boost his private practice. Before long he was told by the university authorities that he was not to use the medical school's name in any writing he did on the subject of food allergy.

The final rupture between Dr Randolph and the academic world came after he had completed a research project on the hormone ACTH. ACTH (adrenocorticotropic hormone) had only recently been isolated by biochemists, and researchers all over the world were keen to find out more about its functions and possible clinical uses. As Randolph was already well known as an allergist he was approached by the Armour Co. pharmaceutical corporation, which held most of the small available stocks of ACTH, and asked if he would like to study the hormone's effect on eosinophils, a class of white blood cells which are involved in the immunological type of allergic response. He felt honoured by this invitation, especially when he learned that supplies of ACTH were so limited that he would be the only doctor in the Chicago area to be given any.

When the medical school staff heard of this, they suggested that he might like to part with a little of the rare substance so they could enter this trendy area of research too. But still smarting from the ban on mentioning the university name in his publications, Randolph turned a deaf ear to their requests. This proved to be the last straw. Shortly afterwards he was kicked out of his teaching job and left to fend for himself in private practice, branded as a pernicious influence and little better than a crank.

Although Ted Randolph did manage to establish a thriving practice, his dismissal did not bode well for the future of ecological medicine. 'In one way it was a good thing, because it freed me from perpetual academic restrictions,' he told me. 'But on the other hand I lost contacts who could have referred patients to me — and young doctors in the area now regarded me as poison.'

Until now Randolph had been little more than an enthusiast applying methods pioneered by others, but he was soon to extend his attention beyond food allergy.

In his field he naturally tended to attract a large proportion of patients who had not been successfully diagnosed and treated by more conventional doctors. He helped plenty with his diets, but there were still many who did not respond even though their ailments sounded quite similar to those caused by food allergies. Fortunately, though, he had adopted a very meticulous approach to taking his patients' histories. Every time they came to see him he would sit at his typewriter and make a record of every little symptom they related and every activity and situation which seemed to make them feel better or worse.

This rather obsessive habit paid handsome dividends in the case of Mrs N. B., a middle-aged lady who had come to him in December 1947 after exhausting the patience of just about every other physician in the city of Chicago.

She told him that ever since she had been a girl she had suffered from perennial rhinitis (running nose), frequent headaches, hives, intermittent sores, chronic fatigue, irritability and nervousness. She had later started to get wheezing fits. Her physical and mental condition was not helped by her social position. She was an attractive white woman, who had outraged her friends and family by marrying a black man; even though he was a surgeon and they were living in the supposedly liberal North, this alliance had resulted in both husband and wife being ostracized by society.

It is not for nothing that Chicago has the nickname of 'the Windy City'. It stands exposed on the edge of the Great Lakes in the middle of a cyclone belt. When the weathermen broadcast a cyclone warning, sensible folk know it is best to stay inside a building with firm foundations and a good roof. One day in 1951 such a warning went out and all Dr Randolph's patients for that day phoned to cancel their appointments — except Mrs N. B., who had already made the long journey into town and decided to stay there until the weather improved.

Though he had been seeing her for nearly four years, Randolph had been quite unable to make her better. He had identified sensitivities to a few foods and to house dust, which gave her the blocked nose, but her more unpleasant symptoms persisted. She kept coming to him because she said he was the only doctor who would still listen to her.

As she was the only patient he was going to see that afternoon he decided to use the time to go through her whole medical history in detail again to look for clues. She was the kind of person who seems to recall past events in the most minute detail, so he was going to have plenty of material to work on.

The first interesting clue she gave was that she always got her asthma attacks and headaches when she was travelling to Chicago by road. Pressing for details as to where en route the symptoms occurred, Randolph found that they coincided with the passage through a part of northwestern Indiana which is thick with oil refineries.

Whenever she stayed in a downtown Chicago hotel she had to insist on having a room above the twentieth floor. If she stayed at street level the wheezes which had begun in Indiana would persist. If she stayed high above the ground they would clear up within day. Moreover, if while driving her car she got caught behind a diesel truck or bus, she knew from past experience that she was so likely to get an acute bronchospasm that she would go to almost suicidal lengths to overtake it. On occasions she had in fact gone into an unconscious stupor at the wheel of the car when caught in a traffice jam. Fortunately this had usually happened when there were other people in the car, though her fellow passengers had never noticed the fumes and had been completely surprised by her fainting.

She then revealed that she had once had a job selling cosmetics but had soon become so ill that she gave it up. In fact she now got severe reactions whenever she tried to wear perfume. If she tried to paint her nails, her eyelids began to itch and she would quickly develop a rash around her eyes.

All this strongly suggested an extreme sensitivity to chemical vapours. But the list of environmental hazards was only just beginning to unroll. She suffered from hay fever which was like that of a pollen allergy, but she got it outside the pollen season. It emerged that the ailment had begun when pine panelling had been put up in her holiday home and regularly recurred when she went there at the same time every year. Christmas was also a bad time — and it turned out that it was the arrival of the Christmas tree into the house which heralded the onset of symptoms.

She did not need Dr Randolph's detective work to help her identify some of the other chemicals which made her miserable. A whiff of enamel paint, turpentine, lacquer, shellac, varnish or synthetic alcohol could be as bad as a lungful of exhaust fumes. She related that she had thrown out her gas cooker several years earlier because she suspected that its vapours were doing her no good. She felt ill if she went near foam rubber and certain plastics and no longer had these materials in her home: but she would begin to wheeze if she went into another house with gas fires or if she inadvertently slept on a bed with a foam mattress.

Dr Randolph soon became aware from her account that his method of identifying food allergies was shot full of holes. Not only had he been neglecting atmospheric pollution as a possible source of his patients' ills, but he had completely overlooked the chemical contamination in the foods they were testing. Mrs N.B. had told him that she had thrice fallen into a stupor after drinking the sweet green liqueur *crème de menthe*. Other artificially coloured foods — maraschino cherries, commercially prepared mint sauce, frankfurters, cake and pie fillings, jams, sweets, pink ice-cream, to name but a few — could all be tied in with her symptoms.

While she had been doing her elimination diets they had found that tomatoes seemed to make her sick on some occasions but not on others. They soon realized that fresh tomatoes from her own garden were quite all right — but they were still left with a puzzle because her headaches and wheezes resulted from eating some but not all canned tomatoes. After further research it appeared that only tomatoes in lined cans were to blame; those preserved in plain metal cans or glass did her no harm.

When they had first tested beef to see whether it caused a reaction, she had suffered acute asthma and headache, yet she later found that she was quite able to eat beef which had been raised on a neighbour's farm. But this beef was of a kind which was becoming hard to get hold of then and is almost unobtainable today: the animals were not fed commercially processed foods nor injected with antibiotics and the meat had not been treated with anything after slaughtering. The beef she had taken during the feeding tests was bought in the normal way through a butcher, and whenever she took this commercially produced meat again, she got acute symptoms.

Through Mrs N.B., Dr Randolph discovered further lacunae in his old methods of diagnosis and treatment. When he had first incriminated house dust as one of her allergens, he had had one of the dustier-looking chairs sprayed with a product called Dust Seal, which is a hydrolyzed mineral oil. Unfortunately, whenever she now sat on this chair she began to wheeze. She had also reacted badly to an injection of house dust extract of the sort then prepared by drug companies for densitization therapy. Randolph later found that the extract contained phenol, which was apparently used as a preservative. She did not react to a different, phenol-free extract. (Incidentally, it is now known that the allergen in house dust is almost always a tiny bug, the house dust mite, which feeds on dead human skin. We slough off small scales of skin all the time, and mites tend to accumulate in bedrooms, where it is dark, warm and there is a good supply of skin. Over the years a variety of fibres and spores found in house dust were blamed as the common allergen, and the dust mite escaped attention for so long because it was very small, transparent and tended to be carried away on the surface of the liquid used for preparing dust extracts. However, every gram of dust on the average bedroom floor contains more than 100 mites, while a gram of dust from the mattress contains almost 1,500. Injectable extracts containing house dust mites are now manufactured for densitization therapy.)

The list of substances which provoked symptoms was apparently endless; aspirin, ether , saccharin, heavily chlorinated or sulphurous water, refined sugar and many synthetic drugs as well as all foods which had sometime been sprayed with insecticides were inculpated and evey attempt made to remove them from her environment.

But this was not to be a story of miracle cure. The lady seemed to have an ineradicable propensity for becoming sensitive to hidden chemicals in the environment and she remained a cripple. Although it would be unwise to draw any fixed conclusions from such a 'hard case', Mrs N.B. had nevertheless opened Randolph's eyes to a host of health hazards which had barely been considered before. Everybody knew that such chemicals were universally poisonous in large enough doses, but no one had considered that certain individuals might be hypersensitive to tiny quantities.

His new interest in the chemical environment also yielded insights into the mechanism of allergy. One women patient, for instance, had found herself suffering more than ever from asthma and bronchitis after moving into a new home.

Within a few months her complaints had multiplied: she began to suffer from headaches, depression and fainting fits, and got so stiff in her joints and muscles that she had to be helped from chairs.

It was not until almost six months had gone by that a major leak was discovered in her gas cooker. It had apparently been steadily emitting fumes into the kitchen ever since it had been installed. During this time she had got into a strange habit of deliberately opening the door of the oven when it was alight, and inhaling large drafts of the hot air. Whenever she did this she got immediate relief from her asthma. But the benefits only lasted a short time, so she felt tempted to do it more and more often.

This patient was eventually brought to Dr Randolph by her brother four years later. Her mental symptoms and cramp pains had grown worse and worse; she kept falling into a kind of stupor which made the hospital staff think she was a drug addict. Her family was eventually told that she should be committed to an asylum — but her brother drew the line at this and sought out Randolph as a last resort. It was only when he began taking her detailed history that the significance of gas came out. It emerged that the only time she felt really better was when she left Illinois for Arizona and spent a lot of time outside in the sun. Her family had assumed that the sun was doing her good, but Randolph came to a different conclusion. He learned that her house in Arizona had gas-fired heating, a gas cooker and a gas water heater, and that any improvement in her health lapsed when she was kept indoors by bad weather. The good thing about the sun was that it got her outside into the fresh country air and encouraged her to turn off the heating.

Tracing her history back to childhood he found that she had always been 'jittery, irritable and clumsy' and prone to rhinitis, headaches and car sickness. He also found that her childhood home had been heated with kerosene stoves, illuminated by kerosene lamps and that the cooking was done on a kerosene range. She told him that even as a little girl she had preferred being outdoors, where there was 'more air', and that she never felt happier and healthier than when she was away at summer camp.

A sceptical reader who is attuned to conventional medical attitudes might say that Randolph was rash to conclude that these last two cases were definitely the result of chemical allergy. Doctors are generally very wary of patients, especially if they are women, who have a long history of mental upsets and who are prone to vague aches and pains about the body. Both these women were already chronic invalids when he first saw them and he never managed to cure them completely. It is a widely held belief that patients like this adopt a 'sick role'; in other words, they learn that by being ill, or by pretending to be ill, they can attract attention to themselves. Eventually their illness becomes like a crutch to a man with one leg: they feel they cannot go anywhere without it. Their aches and pains, which usually appear to have no obvious physical cause, make the doctor suspect that they are shamming or that they are 'neurotic' or 'hysterical'.

Now, the mind may well be a powerful force for sickness and for health; but terms like neurosis and hysteria are not so much diagnoses as admissions of defeat. All they tell us is that the doctor is baffled. Although a psychiatrist might attempt to find out why the patient should have got into this state in the first place, even his chances of finding a cure would be minimal.

When Dr Randolph called in a neurologist to witness one of the woman's stupors, the specialist's report ended with these words: 'Cataleptic attack. I would strongly suspect hysteria.' This was the most he could suggest from examining the patient. But it was Randolph, who spent as much time examining the patient's environment as the patient herself, who noticed that the attacks consistently followed an exposure to gas.

There was one aspect of her behaviour which particularly intrigued him, though. It was her habit of deliberately inhaling hot air from her gas oven, which made her feel temporarily better. This reminded him of Francis Hare's carbohydrate addicts who raided the larder to slave off their carbohydrate hangover, and of Herbert Rinkel's patients with masked allergy who actually got a 'lift' when they ate the allergenic food regularly.

This phenomenon seemed bizarre and inexplicable — until he found he could tie it in with the new theories about stress which were being propounded by the Canadian physiologist Professor Hans Selye.

Stress does not just mean the 'pressure' to which ambitious and aggressive professionals are supposed to be constantly subjected these days. In medical terms stress is any influence which upsets the body's natural smooth running. To function efficiently every creature needs to be able to maintain an internal equilibrium no matter what is going on in the world around it. But stresses like injury, starvation, heat, cold, disease and emotions can put excessive demands on the system and knock it off its even keel.

In his famous experiments in the 1930s Professor Selye found that animals exposed to stress in the form of cold, injury, poison or violent exercise went through three quite distinct stages of reaction. The first stage was rather like the physical shock reaction many people get after an accident or injury, when blood pressure and body temperature drop dramatically. If the stress was not applied for long, the animal would return to normal quite quickly. If it persisted, however, the animal would begin to adapt itself to it. Selye noticed that if he continued to expose the animals to cold, sublethal doses of drugs or regular physical insults they would learn to put up with them for very long periods. But just when it was beginning to look as if they had permanently adapted themselves to this stressful life-style, the animals would go into a rapid decline and die.

Selye repeated these experiments many times and his observations were matched by similar work done by other researchers. Invariably the animals would move from the 'alarm' reaction of stage one, to the second (adapting) stage and then on to the final stage, exhaustion. If an animal which had reached the adaptive stage was taken out and freed from the stress for a few days its adaptations would disappear. If it was re-exposed to the stress it would go through the whole process again, starting with the alarm reaction of stage one.

As a physiologist Selye was particularly interested in changes in his animals' body chemistry. He found that adaptation was associated, among other things, with the production of vast quantities of the corticosteroid hormones. These hormones are vital for mobilizing the resources which keep the system functioning efficiently: they stimulate glucose production, organize the distribution of fats, fight inflammation and keep an eye on the critical balance between sodium and potassium which facilitates the electrical activity of nerves. By the time his animals had reached stage two the adrenal glands, which manufacture corticosteroids, had swollen enormously to cope with the demand. Eventually the effort would prove too much: the adrenal glands would pack up, leaving the animal unable to resist any further.

Pondering Selye's studies, Ted Randolph began to see a parallel between the stages of the stress reaction and the way his patients behaved. The initial alarm reaction to stress was really very like the anaphylaxis experienced by someone who was acutely allergic to a food he or she only ate occasionally. Moreover, Selye himself had suggested that the alarm reaction was very likely triggered by the release of large amounts of histamine from damaged tissue. As histamine was also involved in acute allergic reactions, the link between the two phenomena looked much tighter.

Selye's second, or adaptive, stage seemed to fit in very well with the idea of masked allergy. Randolph believed that many patients had a basic intolerance for certain foods or chemicals, but because their early reactions were delayed or not violent enough to warn them away from further exposure, they would go on taking them. They would not lose their intolerance but they would adapt themselves to it. Before long they would have come to regard their adapted state as 'normal'. This meant that if they happened to avoid the food or chemical for a day or two they would feel odd because their system was taking the opportunity to revert back to its original, pre-adapted state. If they managed to persist with their abstinence for several days they would actually get right back to this pre-adapted state. This is what Rinkel had done when he gave up eggs; the only trouble was that his next exposure to an egg threw him violently into a stage one 'alarm' reaction. Usually, however, an adapted patient would come to enjoy the 'kick' or 'lift' the food gave him — blithely unaware that this was another sign of the tax he was imposing on his adaptive resources. Eventually these resources would become depleted, and it was then, just as they began to slip into the exhaustion of Selye's third stage, that the severe symptoms of chronic disease would start coming through.

The great problem for the doctor, Randolph reflected, was that he usually first saw his patients when they had already reached the latter stages of adaptation and were beginning to fail. In other words, he was faced with patients who were almost beyond help while millions of others who could easily be helped were running around undiagnosed. Randolph was convinced that allergies were created in the cradle. Eggs, milk and cereals — the commonest allergens — were among the first foods an infant received. Many children made it plain with demonstrations of diarrhoea and colic that they could not tolerate them, but again and again he had heard mothers proudly tell how her child had 'grown out' of its allergy when she had kept on feeding the same food — having been encouraged to do so by his colleagues. Individuals who managed to escape being pushed into a masked allergy during childhood were exposed to a chemical environment over which they had diminishing control and which filled their lungs, mouths and skins with hostile hidden substances. When Randolph expressed his beliefs publicly he was accused of scaremongering. 'Hard cases,' he was told, 'make bad laws.'

3
Environments: The One We Inhabit and the One We Inherit

Chemical Environment

Marks and Spencer's yogurts were wonderful. In fact they were the only yogurts worth eating — as long as you never went near the strawberry-flavoured ones. That was Liz's opinion, and it was an opinion formed by bitter experience with other commercial yogurts.

Liz was first referred to the allergy clinic at London's St Mary's Hospital after a series of doctors had failed to find the cause of the terrible rashes she got after eating all kinds of foods. A minute or two after putting the food to her mouth her lips would swell, and a little later she would have hives appearing all over her body.

The only clear common factor between the foods which made Liz suffer was that they were all packaged or processed. She had also found that one or two of the medicines she had been prescribed over the years gave her the rash too. A survey of the guilty products did not throw suspicion on any particular food ingredient, so the allergist decided to test her reactions to a few of the better-known chemical additives.

It turned out that Liz was allergic to hydrobenzoic acid, a chemical which is widely used as a preservative to stop moulds growing on foods and also as a flavouring agent, especially in sweet foods and drinks. It is therefore popular with yogurt manufacturers, whose products are especially prone to develop moulds. At the time Marks and Spencer's yogurts did not have this additive, so Liz could eat them quite happily. When they added strawberry-flavour yogurt to their range she was keen to try it — but she soon realized her mistake. When the manufacturers subsequently got her phone call telling them that strawberry was not the only new ingredient in their yogurt, they promptly admitted that the preservative had been added too. 'But how *did* you know?' they asked.

If acute reactions to chemical additives were common, the offending substances would soon give themselves away. But Liz's allergy is unusual and without specialist help she might never have pinned it down. Indeed, many doctors might have been tempted to regard her rashes as a nervous reaction, for things like this undeniably can be brought on by emotional upsets in some people, whether they are allergic or not. British medical officialdom has apparently not worried itself in the least about hydrobenzoic acid: as well as going into foods it is a permitted additive in about 250 prescribed and over-the-counter medicines.

In 1948 the American physician Dr Stephen Lockey identified tartrazine as the direct cause of asthma or urticaria in some of his patients. Tartrazine is a yellow dye used commonly in processed foods. Dr Lockey had not been testing his patients for food allergy; he had noticed that they reacted allergically to the medicines he was prescribing for them, and eventually realized that the only possible culprit was the colouring material. Tartrazine is added to some drugs as a preservative, though more often it is used purely as a colouring and flavouring agent to make the medicine more acceptable to the patient who has to take it.

It took another thirty years of painstaking investigation and documentation of adverse reactions to tartrazine for Dr Lockey to convince the American Government and drug companies that tartrazine was probably doing considerable harm and very little good. Manufacturers in the United States have now agreed to a voluntary ban of tartrazine in most medicines, but in Britain the chemical has been used in about two hundred medical preparations and in countless foods, including some of anti-inflammatory drugs and tranquillizers which are prescribed in tens of millions every year.

Admittedly, not everyone who takes these drugs is breaking out in a rash or getting asthma, but it is ironic that tartrazine should be added to several medicines used to treat allergic diseases, and is therefore being given to the very people most likely to react to it. The British Committee on the Safety of Medicines has grudgingly recognized the hazards of tartrazine by banning its use in new medicines designed for allergic people. But medicines introduced before 1978 which contain tartrazine have not been restricted.

Dr Bill Frankland, the leading British allergist, has had patients whose allergic symptoms got worse after taking Piriton, an antihistamine drug which came in yellow tablets, and Ventolin tablets, which contain a pink colouring and are used for treating asthma. Some patients of his who were thought to have an allergy to penicillin in fact only had adverse reactions when they took yellow penicillin tablets coloured with tartrazine. 'Very few doctors who were not allergy specialists would be aware of this hazard,' he told me. His colleague Dr Bernard Freedman, when working at King's College Hospital, London, found that tartrazine presented a problem in about one of ten of his asthma patients. They would wheeze after taking almost any food coloured with the dye, but their allergy to tartrazine often came to light when they drank orange squash. Natural orange juice would cause them no problem at all, but the coloured squash made them wheeze. Fortunately more publicity has been given to tartrazine in the past few years and medicine manufacturers have begun to eradicate the colour from many of their products.

Allergic patients also have to be warned against wine, which contains sulphur dioxide, one of the most potent chemicals known to cause allergic reactions. Most soft drinks contain sulphur dioxide and/or benzoic acid, which is also sometimes an allergen.

Oriental gourmets have their own allergy, known as the Chinese Restaurant syndrome. One evening in 1969 a Chinese-American doctor, Robert Kwok, was dining out in his favourite Chinese restaurant when he was stricken with 'numbness at the back of the neck, radiating to both arms and the back, with general weakness and palpitations.' He thought he had had a heart attack, and was admitted to a hospital as an emergency case. Investigations at the hospital showed that he had not had the suspected coronary, however, and his symptoms had by then disappeared. But a few weeks later the same thing happened. This time he was sure it was a heart attack and was whisked off to the hospital once more. Again it was shown that his heart was functioning normally. Finally it dawned on him that both attacks had occurred in the same restaurant just after he had finished his meal.

When he described his experience to friends and colleagues he learned that several had had similar attacks — and always after eating a Chinese meal. He eventually worked out that the cause of the Chinese Restaurant syndrome was monosodium glutamate, a flavouring agent derived from soya beans or wheat which is widely used in Chinese cooking. When he reported this to the *New England Journal of Medicine,* several other doctors sent in their own accounts of patients suffering the same thing in similar circumstances.

The principal concern of government agencies towards additives is that they should not cause cancer. No other disease evokes such strong emotion as cancer and this is the main reason why politicians have wanted to be seen as crusaders against this plague. In 1958 the US Government amended its food and drug laws by adding the Delaney clause, which stated that 'No additive shall be deemed safe if it is found to induce cancer when ingested by man or animal'. The Delaney clause was directly responsible for, among other things, the ban on cyclamate sweeteners. But there are a number of substances which have escaped being banned because no one has proved they cause cancer, even though they may cause other diseases. Nitrates and nitrites are examples. Sodium nitrite and nitrate are used by meat-packaging companies as a preservative and colour fixer to prevent meats losing their redness. Once eaten they can combine with the body's acids to produce nitrosamines, some of which can cause tumours. Nitrites get into rivers, and thence into the water supply, from 'treated' sewerage and from farmers' fields which have been sprayed with nitrogen-based fertilizers. In this case it is babies who are most at risk: high levels of nitrites in local water supplies have been seen to coincide with minor epidemics of the blue baby syndrome in infants under six months old who are being bottle fed. The chemical damages haemoglobin, and this prevents the blood from carrying sufficient oxygen.

In June 1978 Mr Norman Nicholson, a scientist working for the Thames Water Authority, disclosed to an international meeting that nitrate levels in the rivers which supplied London's drinking water exceeded the World Health Organization's safety limit of 11.3 milligrams a litre for up to 'several weeks at a time'. The problem was particularly bad in summer, when there was less water in the rivers to dilute the constant supply of sewage and agricultural effluent. Although filtering techniques were able to remove a certain amount, water which was 'over the limit' did sometimes reach

Londoners' taps. The problem has been most acute in East Anglia, where water authorities have had to send uncontaminated bottled water to certain homes with young babies when the nitrate levels get too high. In certain agricultural areas of the northern United States where there is no piped water supply, residents have little option but to use well water which contains three or four times the recommended maximum of nitrates. Fertilizers are largely to blame for this, and these high concentrations of nitrates are found in water draining from arable land which is regularly sprayed.

Perhaps the most intimate way of demonstrating the inroads chemicals have made into our diet is to examine a piece of bread and butter. Fifty years ago a homemade loaf from a country kitchen would have been made from wheat flour, yeast, salt and water, perhaps with a little egg and milk. The butter would have been pure cream, possibly with a pinch of salt. A standard white supermarket loaf today could contain, allowing for small variations between manufacturers, the following:

refined wheat flour
milk
egg
yeast
water
preservatives (a choice of about ten in regular use)
lard (from pork)
vegetable oil (corn, peanut, sunflower, etc.)
calcium propitionate (to prevent moulds)
salt, with added iodine
sugar
synthetic vitamins (niacin, riboflavin, thiamine)
benzoyl peroxide bleach
tricalcium phosphate (to make flour run smoothly)
potassium bromate maturing agent

The additives towards the end of the list may only account for one part in six hundred of the total weight, but of course most people eat bread every day, and a lifetime's exposure might come to more than fifty pounds. As well as these we have to take account of residues of herbicides, insecticides and even dead insects ground up with the wheat.

The butter will contain synthetic hormones (from the cow's diet), yellow butter dye, penicillin, added minerals and synthetic vitamins, fish oil, citrus juice and alcohol solvent.

Then we must not forget that the bread was baked in a pan which had been washed with detergents, and oiled to let the cooked product drop out more easily. The bread wrapper and the milk carton will have absorbed all the chemicals used in their manufacture, as well as waxes and inks. If the bread comes in a clear wrapper, the cellophane or plastic will be gradually releasing synthetic gases trapped in them since they came off the production line.

All or any of these ingredients could present a threat to health; but while it is comparatively easy to identify allergic reactions to the natural organic foods like wheat, milk and eggs, we can only speculate about the chemicals. The conventional method for testing whether a chemical is fit for human consumption is to feed it to healthy laboratory animals and observe whether they sicken. In Britain £50 million a year is spent this way by the government and the food and drug industry, though the value of all this effort and expense is debatable. In 1978 Britain's most prestigious scientific association, the Royal Society, issued a report on the methods currently used for assessing the long-term risks to exposure to drugs and chemicals. The experts who contributed to this report had widely differing opinions about many matters, but they did basically concur that conventional tests were of limited value.

On the one hand, they commented, it was possible to raise unnecessary alarm by drawing ominous conclusions from tests which exposed animals to situations far more extreme than anything a human would have to endure. 'We have only a very crude idea whether a chemical found to be carcinogenic [cancer-causing] in a particular model system would prove a real risk in practice,' the experts admitted.

On the other hand, they pointed out, a great many experiments were performed simply because they were the routine required by law; the researchers would just note the effects of the chemical on the animal and make no attempt to find out how this effect was brought about.

The report's most significant conclusion, however, was that

nutrition and other factors which make some individuals highly susceptible to adverse reactions were 'poorly understood and little studied'.

The need for some kind of official control of mass-produced foods first became apparent in the nineteenth century, when food adulteration was commonplace. Some of the tricks were relatively harmless — the 'sawdust in the sausage meat' variety. Others were horrifying: dill pickles were made greener with copper sulphate; alum was added to flour; lead salts were used to colour cheeses; and sulphuric acid was used by brewers to make their beer mature quickly. The main aim of the antiadulteration laws passed before 1900 was to discourage manufacturers from deliberately poisoning their consumers.

For a few years it seemed as though the pure food lobby would prevail. In 1906 the US Government passed a Pure Food and Drugs Act, which was intended to ensure that toxic substances were not foisted upon the public, and provided for the investigation of all chemical additives by official scientists. Much of the momentum for the act had come from Dr Harvey W. Wiley, chief of the Bureau of Chemistry in the US Department of Agriculture, who had persuaded a dozen healthy young male volunteers to take part in a long-term assessment of the risks presented by food preservatives in common use. They were prescribed balanced diets based on popular foods, so designed that the volunteer was exposed to just one of the preservatives for a long period. They were then regularly measured, weighed and medically examined. Wiley's volunteers attracted the nickname 'the Poison Squad' and their gallantry was widely praised in the press. After a few years Wiley had collected much evidence to suggest that his volunteers had not thrived on their diets, and he declared all the common preservatives — benzoic acid, sulphur dioxide, formaldehyde, salicylic acid and boracic acid — to be bad for the health.

His campaign had no lasting effect, however. The food manufacturers quickly learned how to use the new laws to their advantage. The standards which had been laid down were geared to eliminating the more obvious poisons and adulterants, but made little provision for the accumulative effects of tiny amounts of chemicals over many years. The validity of Wiley's Poison Squad evidence was challenged. The manufacturers also persuaded the authorities that preservatives not only made commercial sense, but political and economic sense too. Not everybody, they pointed out, lived on an ample farm where fresh food was always at hand. Food had to be transported, stored, sold and resold a number of times before it reached an urban household. If there were not preservatives there would be wastage, and that was something the country could not afford.

It is harder to apply this logic to colours and flavours, but in this field food and drug manufacturers have courted public tastes rather than pay attention to real needs. We do not need for instance, to eat yellow butter, or to insist on blush-coloured bacon. Yellowness in butter and redness in bacon have been mistakenly associated with creaminess and freshness, and manfacturers found that foods with the 'right' colour sold best. So as long as they kept within the law the obvious commercial answer was to endow their product with the hue most people seemed to want.

(Colouring and flavouring are a little more justifiable in medicines. A sweet taste may be the only way a mother can get a child to take a bitter pill, and a distinctive colour may prevent an unfortunate old person from confusing his heart pill with his laxative. Colour may even have some therapeutic value; in 1974 the *British Medical Journal* reported that patients given green pills felt significantly better for their treatment than patients given the same drug in red pills!)

By seeking to please the customer, food technology has finally succeeded in disorienting and deceiving him. Brown sugar and brown flour were orginally just the unrefined version of white sugar and white flour. They were purchased for their flavour and their wholesomeness. But today anyone who goes out to buy brown sugar or brown flour has to be careful lest he is sold white sugar which has been coloured with molasses or white flour which has been dyed brown. (The British sugar refiners Tate & Lyle had a long legal battle over the use of the term 'demerara sugar'. They were finally told that they could not call white sugar treated with molasses demerara, but they were allowed to label it 'London Demerara'.) Most of the asparagus eaten today is canned and has a slightly metallic taste. So many consumers have come to regard this taste as normal that some American food packers who pack their asparagus in glass jars took to adding metal salts to give it the familiar taste.

To be fair to the manufacturers, they are arguably just as much victims of their technology as the consumers. According to a report from the British Government's Food Additives and Contaminants Committee published in March 1979, a leading manufacturer lost 50 per cent of its sales when it removed the added colouring from its canned peas and strawberry jam. The manufacturer therefore put a little colouring back into those products, but still took two years to recover the lost customers.

About three thousand synthetic and natural chemicals are now used for preserving, colouring, flavouring and stabilizing prepared foods. Unless we adopt Arthur Coca's lunchbox technique and refuse to eat anything which is not grown on our very own unpolluted organic acres, we can hardly avoid eating about four pounds of these unsolicited substances every year. In sufficiently large doses many would be indisputably poisonous, but we do not eat large quantities very quickly. Some chemicals act synergistically, that is to say they produce a much stronger reaction when they are together than they can by themselves. Alcohol and barbiturates are a well-known example of drugs which act this way, often with fatal consequences.

In California researchers working for the US Department of Agriculture devised a method for preserving uncooked cut potatoes by immersing them in a refrigerant called difluourodichloromethane, better known as Freon 12. The potatoes were then steeped in tepid water, fried very lightly, refrozen and subsequently sold in supermarkets. The justification for this chemical assault was an alleged public demand for instant french fries with a better taste and texture than the partly cooked brands previously available.

The Food and Drug Administration, the government agency charged with enforcing the food and drug laws, had approved Freon 12, which is a chemical cousin of dry-cleaning fluid, as being fit for such culinary applications. As usual, the decision had been based on studies of the chemical's effect, alone, on healthy animals. It was not until some years later that the scientific journal *Nature* reported that a common ingredient of pesticides, piperonyl butoxide, acted synergistically with Freons, and that the combination had proved lethal and carcinogenic in mice.

Considering the popularity of pesticides and instant french fries in California, it is reasonable to assume that somebody, some time, has been exposed to this cancer cocktail. A light exposure has to be considered in the context of countless other exposures to combinations of chemicals about which we know very little. You never know — the fact that we are all still alive may just be due to unknown *beneficial* synergistic reactions which make up for the damage done by the rest.

Even with drugs, which have been subjected to much more scrutiny than food chemicals, no one has produced an infallible method for predicting dangerous side-effects. The long-term effects of the hormone diethylstilboestrol, which was widely prescribed in the 1950s to prevent mothers miscarrying, only manifest themselves a generation later, when some of these mothers' daughters developed vaginal cancers in their teens. In Britain the thalidomide disaster led to a much tighter system for controlling the development and prescription of new drugs. But these controls did not prevent the brain haemorrhages which befell patients who happened to eat cheese while taking certain antidepressant drugs, nor the severe eye and irreparable gut damage which crippled a few of the many thousands of patients who had been prescribed the heart drug practolol. Even by the most exacting contemporary standards these reactions had been unforeseeable and only came to light when the medicines had been widely used for some years.

When the Royal College of Physicians in London invited a conference of experts to discuss this issue in the wake of the practolol affair in 1976, one of their main conclusions was that patients should accept the risks of medicine as well as its benefits. This advice may be reasonable, always assuming that your doctors are honest, sober, well informed and regard you as something more precious than a laboratory rat. If you are sick and cannot help yourself, the risks are worth taking.

But can we say the same of the deal on offer at the supermarket? Here the chemical technologists present us with plenty of proven risks (nitrites, dyes, preservatives, insecticides, weed killers) and some potential risks we can only speculate about. And of course they offer us benefits (pretty colours, strong flavours, long-life cans, precooking, ease of preparation). In the process they have lost half the natural vitamins, oils and trace elements and at least 10 per cent of the natural protein from their principal staple ingredient, wheat flour. To make up for this, they have added sugar (which we do not need but have developed a taste for), salt (which may well be harming our kidneys and raising our blood-pressure, but which does make all the peas in a can swell conveniently and attractively to exactly the same size) and monosodium glutamate (very tasty, but don't forget Dr Kwok). But the stangest thing they have done is to mix everything up so we no longer know what to expect in the packet. You will be lucky to find apple sauce, tomato sauce, gravy, soup, jam or spreads which do not contain at least 20 per cent wheat or corn starch. Those nuts in the 'nutty' cookies may in fact not be nuts but toasted oats. Corn and wheat have got into instant coffee to keep its price down, and have crept into less reliable brands of ground coffee too. Pea flour may be about to join the old-fashioned wheat flour in your bread.

Milk is almost universal in processed foods in one form or another. As lactose (milk sugar) it is a favourite with bakers and confectioners, and it is used to carry flavourings. People who are milk-allergic should keep an eye open for sodium caseinate, which does not sound like milk but is in fact a milk product. Sodium caseinate really does appear where you would least expect it, namely in 'non-dairy creamer', the milk substitute. Eggs, one of the commonest allergens, are just as widespread, and here too the allergic patient must learn the food trade jargon if he wants to identify egg-based ingredients listed on a food label. The words to look out for are albumin, globulin, ovomucin, ovomucoid, livetin, ovovitellin, vitellin and lecithin. Meanwhile eggs are being ousted from the places we have traditionally expected to find them: in pastries and cakes they are being replaced by variable proportions of vegetable oils, extruded soya bean, corn syrup and peanut flour.

An intriguing newcomer is a yeast brought to us by the Amoco Food Company. Although it has been advertised in food trade journals as a 'natural food ingredient' it is in fact cultured on ethyl alcohol originating from Amoco's oil refineries. Its destination is the meat pie market, where it is apparently popular for its ability to prevent moisture (=weight=profits) oozing out of the product.

It has also been promoted as a cheap alternative to egg yolks and milk solids.

In his remarkable book *Food for Nought* Professor Ross Hume Hall, head of biochemistry at McMaster University in Canada, pointed out that the mushroom growth of food technology has coincided with a decline in the popularity of nutrition as an academic science. Since the Second World War nutrition has failed to attract the 'high flyer' university scientists, he claims. Having almost come to a halt since the discovery of vitamins, the specialty has been quite unable to provide disinterested research into the manufacturing activities of commercial food processors. As a result of this academic stagnation there have been few authoritative voices to counter the propaganda of an industry which has sold American parents and teachers the idea that a doughnut with added vitamin C should be given to schoolchildren for their breakfast because it contains more 'essential nutrients' than fresh fruit.

Nutritionists, Professor Hall says, have become preoccupied with the chemical structure of food and devote little thought to its biology. As an example of the way nutritionists have got out of touch with food technology, he cites an experiment done in 1973 by Dr P. A. Lachance of Rutgers University on chicken pot pies, a frozen food sold in supermarkets for reheating at home. According to the US Department of Agriculture's handbook on the composition of foods, which is the North American dietitian's bible, these pies contained quite a lot of vegetables and should have been full of vitamin C. In fact they contained none. So Lachance added vitamin C to a defrosted pie, put it back in the freezer for two days, and then heated it in the recommended fashion. When the pie was analysed again a quarter of the vitamin C he had added had vanished too.

It is easy to overlook the fact that food processing does not end at the factory. The process continues while the food is being stored in the freezer and prepared in the kitchen. The final stage occurs in the consumer's stomach. It is therefore very difficult to know what we eat and what good or harm we can really expect from our food.

In the 1940s Dr Ted Randolph refined his elimination diets after noticing patients who were sensitive to corn and corn flour also appeared to react badly to sugar and spirits made from corn.

Alcoholic beverages are not highly refined, so it is not very surprising perhaps to find that corn liquor gave them symptoms. Refined sugars, however, were believed to be chemically identical, whatever their origin. His work aroused the interest of the Sugar Research Foundation, whose research director, Dr Hockett, offered to supply him with samples of a glucose of known origin which he could use in feeding tests. Some weeks later a packet arrived at Dr Randolph's office from Cambridge, Massachusetts, containing the promised samples but with no covering letter to explain what the sugar had been made from. Knowing the beet was not grown anywhere within several hundred miles of Cambridge he assumed that it was derived from the imported cane usually processed in East Coast refineries. He subsequently asked nine patients who had previously reacted to particular sugars to help him in an experiment. Three were corn-sensitive, three were cane-sensitive and three were beet-sensitive, and they had only ever reacted to sugar made from the food to which they were allergic. In the experiment each was fed under the tongue with just fifty milligrams of the glucose. Shortly afterwards the three beet-sensitive patients broke out in hives, while the others experienced no physical or mental reaction at all.

Dr Hockett was amazed by Randolph's report. He confirmed that the glucose had come from sugar beet, but pointed out that not even a chemist could have worked this out by analysing the samples he had sent.

Randolph concluded that some allergenic element must remain in the most refined products. He drew support for this theory from his observations of the effects of alcoholic drinks on his patients. At first he had not been able to understand why patients who were allergic to corn and who avoided corn in their diet should get their symptoms after drinking a little Scotch whisky or applejack brandy, which were not supposed to contain any corn liquor. He persuaded an Illinois distillery to let him have samples of pure spirits derived from each of the crops used for making liquor. He found that the corn-sensitive patients reacted to the corn alcohol but not to the alcohol made from barley or apples. So why did they react to whisky and applejack? When he put this question to his contacts in the booze trade he learned that much of the whisky exported to the United States had been deliberately 'bourbonized' to make it appeal to American tastes. In other words, corn liquor produced in the United States and elsewhere was imported into Scotland, added to the export whisky, which was then shipped to America. Corn got into applejack in the form of a caramel colouring made from corn and cane sugar.

Randolph's findings were published in medical journals, where they may have raised a few eyebrows. Unfortunately, nobody seems to have been sufficiently intrigued by the implications to repeat the experiments. So while some American allergists follow Randolph's advice and warn their patients to keep off refined sugar, others do not believe that sugar presents any allergic risks.

Randolph also claims that chemical contaminants in sugar produce allergic reactions. He found that patients who reacted badly to sugar made from cane did not suffer any reaction if they ate cane sugar which had not gone through a certain filtering process used in refining. The filters used in the process were made of beef bone char, and they were periodically cleaned by being exposed to an open gas flame at 1000° centigrade. As his patients only reacted to sugar which had been passed through such filters, he assumed that the filters must contain some gas or other chemical contaminant which was being imparted to the sugar.

Although most doctors regard Randolph's preoccupation with chemical contaminants as excessively alarmist, it is undeniable that the tiniest amounts of chemical gases and dusts — or indeed any allergen — can provoke violent reactions in people who are sensitive to them. Platinum salts, for instance, are a common cause of asthma and bronchitis in industrial workers who are regularly exposed to them. Once a sensitivity to these salts has developed, a few molecules can cause a reaction. The standard test for platinum salts sensitivity consists of injecting the skin with a millionth of a gram of a solution which contains one part in a billion of the salts. If the patient is sensitive to these salts, this infinitesimally small dose will make a button-size weal appear on the skin.

Similarly it has been found that factory workers can become sensitive to toluene di-isocyanate, a chemical used in the manufacture of varnishes and adhesives. In test conditions these workers have suffered acute asthma just ten minutes after being exposed to air containing one part in a billion of the chemical.

Not all reactions are so immediate and obvious. Some allergic workers only start to wheeze a few hours after they have been exposed to a particular chemical. Because their symptoms occur when they have gone home after work or when they are in bed at night, it often takes a very long time for a doctor to suspect that the allergen might be in the factory rather than in the home.

Tiny moulds and spores which are only visible under a microscope account for a whole range of occupational diseases. There is farmer's lung, a chest complaint caused by an allergy to moulds which grow on warm, damp hay; malt-worker's lung from moulds on barley and malt; bird-fancier's lung from pigeon and budgerigar droppings; woodworker's lung from sawdust; cheese-washer's lung from cheese mites and moulds; New Guinea lung from mouldy thatch; bagassosis from moulds which grow on rotting sugar cane; and ventilation pneumonitis, an allergy to tiny organisms which populate air-conditioning and ventilation systems. When, as often happens, the disease is not diagnosed in its early stages and the patient continues to be exposed to the offending antigen, it ends up as a chronic inflammation of the lung. Even then the patient's doctor is unlikely to come up with an accurate diagnosis unless he is familiar with such occupational hazards. When doctors at the Cardiothoracic Institute of London, one of the leading research centres on this kind of disease, looked at the medical notes of more than a hundred of their patients suffering from malt-worker's lung they found that more than half had been wrongly diagnosed as tuberculosis, lung cancer or collapsed lung by doctors who had not suspected the presence of an allergen in the patient's workplace.

As many of these occupational diseases have only been identified during the past ten years, we can assume that the search for allergenic spores and gases has only just begun, and that industrial exposures must account for much more sickness and death than we ever suspected before.

Professor Jack Pepys, former Head of the Immunology Department at the Cardiothoracic Institute, has been a pioneer in this field of industrial allergies. In an interview he warned me that we should be cautious about drawing too much attention to unproven hazards: 'By telling someone that he may have a sensitivity to chemicals, you can make him so anxious that he will believe that he has an allergy to every chemical under the sun. All you succeed in doing is to frighten your patients out of their wits, and we have no right to do this.'

Professor Pepys also points out that the symptoms which some doctors ascribe to chemical allergies are 'vague and not easy to measure objectively'. 'There is a great difference, for instance, between an attack of asthma or hives, which is obvious and simple to examine, and the generalized aches and pains and malaises which are hard to examine objectively but which the ecologists attribute to food or chemical allergies.'

On the other hand he concedes that the patients he sees do very often have these vaguer symptoms too, and that it is quite conceivable that certain people may be more prone to psychiatric than physical reactions. There is no rule which confines allergic reactions to the skin or the airways.

The great unsolved problem confronting allergists is why only a minority of people should become sensitive to a particular substance. Some substances, notably platinum salts and castor beans, succeed in sensitizing more than half the people who are regularly exposed to them. These are unusually potent allergens and not every substance has such allergic potential. However, it does seem that the longer you are exposed to a possible allergen, the more likely you are to become sensitized. So far no one has worked out how much exposure is necessary to cause an allergy.

When immunologists began studying patients with farmer's lung they found that these people had large amounts of antibody to hay moulds. Unfortunately this did not offer much of a clue about the way the disease developed, because not long afterwards they also found that any farm worker who had ever been exposed to these moulds would have antibodies too, even though he had no symptoms of the disease. Antibodies to egg, milk and other allergens have been found both in healthy people and allergic people; so it seems that antibodies may only tell us whether a person has been exposed to a substance but do not prove whether or not he or she has an allergy.

Although the immunologists like to define allergy as an abnormal reaction by the immune system, they have found it hard to show that all chemical allergies are activated by antigens and antibodies.

Their search has not been made any easier by the fact that antibodies can only be produced to proteins, which are made up of big molecules. Most industrial chemicals and gases have small molecules, and before they can arouse the attention of the immune system they have to attach themselves to the proteins which are already floating around in the blood or tissues. To distinguish them from the other allergens, these non-protein chemical allergens are called haptens. Antibodies have been found to some hapten/protein combinations, but not to some of the other major chemical allergens, notably aspirin. So it is still not certain whether antibodies are really involved in all chemical allergies.

The Environment We Inherit

In the section on immunology and allergies in Appendix I, I mention that some allergic people appear to lack a 'suppressor cell' which could control the production of antibodies. This could be an inherited defect. Some allergies may be due to the lack of an enzyme, and this deficiency could also be inherited. Enzymes exist to break down proteins and amino acids, so if a particular enzyme is missing, excessive amounts of certain proteins and amino acids may accumulate and spark off inflammations or other reactions. Favism, a type of anaemia which affects Mediterranean peoples who eat fava (broad) beans, only seems to strike those who lack a digestive enzyme which degrades the fava allergen before it reaches the blood-stream.

Some people get terrible stomach cramps, diarrhoea and wind when they drink milk. Though this is often the result of an antibody reaction to milk proteins, it can also be due to a deficiency of lactase, the enzyme which breaks down lactose (milk sugar). Lactase deficiency is much commoner in some races than others. It is rare among white Europeans and Americans, but very common among black people, Japanese and South-east Asian people.

There is also a whole group of diseases which most doctors would regard as completely unrelated to each other but which appear to run in families. They are very relevant to the theme of this book because they are the principal diseases associated with food allergy; asthma, eczema, dyslexia, migraine, coeliac disease, epilepsy and schizophrenia.

Over the years many doctors have pointed out that someone who had one of these diseases was very likely to have a parent or grandparent who suffered from it too. Early in this century the English psychiatrist George Savage noticed that there was an apparent connection between asthma and eczema and mental illnesses. He observed that if schizophrenic or depressed patients in his asylum improved sufficiently to be discharged, they would often begin to suffer from asthmas or eczema once they got home. After a while these symptoms would disappear, only to be replaced by a new bout of their mental illness.

In 1975 Dr Vera Walker, a migraine specialist and former president of the British Association of Allergists, became intrigued by the increasing number of reports from doctors in Britain, the United States and Canada which blamed various mental illnesses as well as migraine and the common allergic complaints like asthma on allergies to food and chemical contaminants. She wondered whether there was any common factor between these diseases.

With the help of the Migraine Association, the Dyslexia Association and other patients' organizations, she sent out a questionnaire to hundreds of families who had at least one member who suffered from migraine, dyslexia, coeliac disease or schizophrenia, asking them whether they had close relatives suffering from the same disease or from any others in the group. By close relatives she meant grandparents, parents, brothers and sisters and children, so the survey covered four generations in each family. Tables II, III, IV and V show the figures she obtained from the replies.

What these figures reveal is that someone who suffers from migraine, dyslexia, coeliac disease or schizophrenia has a far higher than normal chance of having a close relative who suffers from this disease or one of the others listed. Although the figures for epilepsy and the mental illnesses look rather low when we compare them with those for migraine and asthma, they are much higher than what we would expect to find in a survey of these diseases in the general population.

Table II 1,534 migraine families	
Diagnosis	No. of cases in close relatives
MIGRAINE	4,538
asthma	1,058
eczema or urticaria	1,548
dyslexia	210
coeliac	103
epilepsy	256
schizophrenia	86
other mental illness	540

Table II 138 dyslexia families	
Diagnosis	No. of cases in close relatives
DYSLEXIA	256
migraine	336
asthma	128
eczema or urticaria	202
coeliac	9
epilepsy	31
schizophrenia	18
other mental illness	64

Table IV 83 coeliac families	
Diagnosis	No. of cases in close relatives
COELIAC	108
migraine	265
asthma	73
eczema or urticaria	117
dyslexia	7
epilepsy	16
schizophrenia	5
other mental illness	47

Table V schizophrenia families	
Diagnosis	No. of cases in close relatives
SCHIZOPHRENIA	91
migraine	246
asthma	83
eczema or urticaria	104
dyslexia	25
coeliac	22
epilepsy	4
other mental illness	61

Now, while it is very interesting to discover that diseases run in families, this fact does not often help doctors make their patients better. What interested Dr Walker was that all these diseases had also been linked with food allergy. This suggested two things: firstly that some families were more vulnerable to all kinds of allergic disease, and secondly that anyone suffering from any of these diseases should be examined for possible food or chemical allergy before being given the normal treatment for these various diseases, which consisted of being prescribed drugs or packed off to a psychiatric hospital.

Before we move on to look at how allergies are diagnosed and treated we should consider one other important and intimate part of our environment in early life — the breast. As well as feeding the baby, a mother's milk passes on antibodies which protect the baby until its own immunological resources have developed. This explains why breast-fed babies suffer fewer infections than bottle-fed babies. But although breast milk is the ideal food for an infant it can also be a source of allergies. It can carry proteins from foods which the mother has eaten; for instance, breast-fed babies sometimes get rashes or colic after their mother has been eating chocolate, eggs, wheat or milk. When the mother stops taking these foods, the baby recovers. Not every breast-fed child reacts this way to its mother's diet, but those who do tend to come from families with a history of allergy. All foreign proteins are potential allergens, and the more a susceptible child is exposed to them, the greater the chances of it becoming sensitized, perhaps permanently.

I am afraid that we emerge from this chapter with more questions than answers. We know that some chemicals in our food, drink and atmosphere can make us sick, but we do not know why some of us are more vulnerable to allergies than others. We know that some chemicals to which we are exposed can potentiate each other, but the extent of such reactions and their effects on us over a long period are almost completely unknown. We know that the majority of supermarket foods contain hidden allergens which can escape the attention of even the most avid label reader. And although many diseases associated with food and chemical allergies run in families, we do not know exactly what part heredity, diet and infant feeding each play in this process.

Having admitted how little we really know, let's go on to see how food and chemical allergies are diagnosed, treated and prevented.

4

Diagnosis and Desensitization

One summer afternoon in 1960 Dr Herbert Rinkel — the man, you may recall, who thirty years previously had almost been killed by a piece of angel cake — was sitting at the table with a colleague and his wife. Like Rinkel, Dr Carlton Lee had been drawn to the subject of allergy by personal experience. He was allergic to several foods, especially coffee, and his wife had suffered from asthma, which she had only been able to avoid by giving up eating beef. Dr Rinkel knew about his friends' food allergies and was therefore taken aback when he saw Mrs Lee serve beef for lunch and tuck into it with great enthusiam.

'What has happened to your beef allergy, Mrs Lee?' he ventured to ask.

'I still have it,' she replied. 'But thanks to these injections Carlton gives me, it is now quite under control'.

Dr Lee then joined in the conversation to say that he would be taking coffee after lunch. He explained that as long as he took an injection of his specially prepared coffee extract before meals he could now drink the beverage without fear of suffering his old allergic reactions.

These revelations amazed Rinkel. Though he was one of the most enthusiastic proponents of food allergy, this treatment was something quite new. More than thirty years before, allergists had found that if you injected food extracts into patients' skin you could produce all their allergic symptoms. But though many had tried, no one had found a way of curing food allergy with injections.

It was strange that food allergy did not respond to this kind of treatment, because many allergists, including Rinkel himself, had successfully used injection therapy on patients with hay fever and other allergies to pollen and spores. Theoretically, therefore, food allergy should have been treatable this way too, although all attempts to find a method had ended in disappointment.

Carlton Lee explained that he had been experimenting with injections of food extracts into the skin to see what kind of reaction they would cause. He had found that an injection of an extract would produce a weal, whose size depended on the amount of extract injected. The more dilute the extract was, the smaller the weal would be, until you reached a point where no reaction occurred.

What Dr Lee had done was to continue injecting increasingly dilute solutions of food extract. Remarkably, he found that if he went two or three stages of dilution beyond the point where wealing had disappeared, the injection actually relieved the patient's illness. Instead of provoking symptoms, it made them disappear, sometimes for several days. Thus, by trial and error he had eventually worked out how to give patients doses of diluted antigen which could be relied upon to 'switch on' or 'switch off' symptoms.

'And that explains how my wife can eat beef without getting her asthma,' he told Rinkel.

Rinkel was so enthused by Lee's work that he joined him in his research. It was not long before they came across another remarkable phenomenon. They found that if they took their dilutions a few stages further than the switch-off point, injections would start to make the weals reappear. This was not just a freak phenomenon which had happened in one or two patients and could have been the result of error: it occurred consistently and repeatedly. In other words, you could switch on symptoms with a smaller dose than you needed to switch them off.

Lee and Rinkel thus formulated a treatment for food allergy and a method for diagnosing it which has been practised by clinical ecologists ever since. Some prefer to give drops of food sublingually (under the tongue) rather than injections, but the principle is the same. Demonstrations of sublingual switch-ons and switch-offs can be highly dramatic. Five minutes after being given a drop of flour solutions under their tongue, patients who suffer from mental illness may start to cry and quickly become very agitated. Five minutes later, after a neutralizing dose a hundred or perhaps a thousand times more dilute has been administered, they will be as quiet and happy as lambs in spring.

The medical profession in general, however, has regarded these techniques with utter scepticism. The general opinion of doctors who know little else about the theory or practice of clinical ecology, has been that if the treatment works at all it must be due to a placebo response or perhaps even hypnosis.

Admittedly their reservations about these methods are not altogether unjustified. Skin tests work much more reliably on people who have acute, immediate reactions to foods and chemicals than on people whose allergic reactions do not happen for a long time — many hours, sometimes days — after they have eaten the food. This may be because their reactions are caused by different mechanisms: the fast reactors having a Type One allergy sparked off by IgE, while the slow reactors have a Type Four allergy or react for some completely different reason. (See Appendix I for a more detailed explanation of these terms.) And in 1974 the American College of Allergists made its own study of sublingual tests and concluded that they were unreliable.

More recently, though, the allergists who believe in these methods have begun to answer their critics with objective clinical studies of their own. Dr Doris Rapp, a well-known American allergist who lost her job as associate professor at an American university when she persisted in using these controversial methods, has now proved their value in 'double-blind' trials with hyperactive children and mentally disturbed adults who suffer from food or chemical allergy. Dr Marshall Mandell of New York and psychologist Dr David King of the University of Massachusetts have also completed a study which vindicated sublingual testing for food allergy.

In a double-blind trial, neither the doctor nor the patient knows whether the medicine administered is the real thing or an inert substitute. All the pills are made to look alike and each patient's prescription is handed over to the doctor already packed and numbered by a supervisor. It is only after the results of the treatment have been assessed that the supervisor reveals which patients have been getting the real thing and which ones have been getting the placebo. If the patients who were given the real thing have done much better than those who got the placebo, we can assume that the real thing has genuine value.

In Mandell and King's trial thirty patients with at least one psychological problem — depression, anxiety, confusion, persistent irritability or inability to concentrate — were interviewed about their eating habits. If they said they had a craving for a particular food, got a 'lift' from the food, or ever went on a binge, compulsively eating it in large amounts, an extract of that food was prescribed for a sublingual test.

All Mandell did was to draw up a list of foods for each patient. King, who had been assigned to this investigation for his PhD thesis, then made conventional psychological assessments of each patient, noting all the mental and physical symptoms they complained of. It was also his job to administer the drops of extract under each patient's tongue. Every patient went through a total of eighteen provocation tests during the course of the trial, twelve of the challenges being with a real extract and the other six with a placebo of distilled water. To make sure that neither King nor the patients could tell which syringes contained extract and which contained water, they were handed to him in random order with their barrels covered in opaque paper. Two independent professional observers were called in to assess the patients' reactions to each challenge.

As this kind of investigation put the patients in an unfamiliar situation which might have affected their response, the observers were also asked to assess them before they had been challenged, to establish a psychological base rate. It was all so arranged that the observers would not know whether they were assessing a patient who had just received an extract, one who had been given the distilled water or one who had not been challenged at all that day. The patients themselves were asked to assess their mental and emotional reactions to each challenge by recording them on a scale which ran from *one* for a slight reaction to *seven* for a severe reaction. To lend the project more objectivity, both observers also had to agree that a real reaction had occurred if it was to be included in the patient's records.

When the results of this complicated study were decoded and analysed, it became clear that the food challenges had consistently provoked more frequent mental reactions than the distilled water. Statistically the odds against these results being a mere fluke were 150 to 1, which in scientific circles is generally accepted to be reasonable evidence that the therapy works.

The mental reactions to the allergen extracts were also significantly more severe than any reaction elicited by a placebo. The extracts also provoked a greater variety of symptoms; whereas the placebos only managed to evoke symptoms which the patient had already said he was experiencing during the assessment of his or her base rate, the allergens stimulated reactions which the patient had not suffered for some time.

All things considered, the results offered persuasive evidence that psychological symptoms could be provoked by sublingual tests. Admittedly the technique was not foolproof: the fact that distilled water could sometimes cause a reaction meant that the doctor should be aware of relying absolutely on tests for making a diagnosis. But there are few medical tests which do not sometimes give false-positive results.

Interestingly the study showed that sublingual testing was not a very reliable way of provoking *physical* reactions to allergens. It turned out that distilled water was almost as good at bringing on aches and pains, coughs, snuffles and nausea as the food extracts.

Physical symptoms may respond better to injections. In 1977 Dr Joseph Miller of Alabama and his colleagues did a double-blind trial of the skin injection technique which had been pioneered by Carlton Lee. Patients with a variety of recurring and intractable symptoms which had been attributed to food allergy were given switch-off doses of food extracts or a placebo of salt water. The food injections proved to be significantly more effective than the placebos, and symptoms which had persisted for years often disappeared altogether after three or four days. When patients who had been give a placebo were subsequently put on the food extracts, they began to improve too; but patients who were taken off the food injections and given the salt water began to get their old symptoms back after a few days.

Of course, even if we accept that psychological symptoms can be turned on and off by drops of dilute food extract, we still cannot explain why it happens. This phenomenon has not only been noticed by unorthodox food allergists. It has also puzzled orthodox immunologists.

Allergists who treat hay fever have noticed that a patient who is exposed to just a few grains of pollen may react as violently as if he had run into a pollen cloud. But between these extremes there appear to be degrees of exposure which do not bring symptoms on at all.

Dr Jonathan Brostoff, an immunologist at the Middlesex Hospital Medical School in London, has also found that truly minute quantities of pollen applied to a patient's skin in a prick test can cause as strong a reaction as a large quantity. The prick test is a standard method of diagnosing pollen sensitivity. A small drop of solution containing pollen is placed on the forearm, and the skin beneath is then pricked lightly with a needle. If the patient is at all sensitive to the pollen, a weal will appear within minutes. Normally about 10,000 'Noon units', about a hundredth of a gram (these units are named after the allergy pioneer Dr L. Noon, of St Mary's) are used in prick tests. Experimenting with weaker dilutions Dr Brostoff found that test doses containing 1,000, 100 or one unit produced progressively smaller skin reactions. But if the dose was taken as low as 0.0001 of a unit, full-size weals would reappear.

You may also remember from the last chapter that people who develop a sensitivity to platinum salts will react to a few molecules given in a skin test. If reactions were related to dose, we would expect a sensitive person to die from anaphylaxis if exposed to the average amount of dust flying about his workplace. Strangely, though, it does not happen in quite such a straightforward fashion.

A new drug, levamisole, which is being used experimentally to boost the immune system for the treatment of certain chronic diseases, appears to work as well in tiny doses as in large doses, though doses in between these levels are ineffective. Why? Nobody knows.

Some doctors only use sublingual tests for diagnosing allergies. If the patient reacts — reactions differ widely and include racing pulse, headache, weeping, dilating or contracting pupils, agitation or sleepiness — the symptom is promptly switched off with a lower dose. The patient is then advised to avoid the food or chemical in question and given guidance about diets and ways of avoiding foods.

Others use sublinguals or intradermal injections as treatment. The great disadvantage of this treatment is that the switch-off only lasts for a day or two. This is fine for the manufacturer or doctor in private practice who knows that his customers will have to keep coming back for more extracts, but it may prove expensive to the patient. On the other hand, if it works it does save you from the inconvenience of having to follow an exclusion diet, and does allow you to eat away from home in places where you cannot be certain what hidden allergens the food contains.

Desensitization Methods

Late one night a few years ago Dr Bill Frankland was called from his bed by a telephone call. On the other end of the line was a young doctor on night duty at St Mary's Hospital. 'That patient you discharged a couple of days ago, the one with the allergy to fish. He's just been admitted as an emergency — anaphylaxis.'

This unfortunate fellow (he did survive, incidentally) had first come to St Mary's for help after a disagreeable experience with his girl friend. He had always been acutely allergic to fish and had tried his best to keep away from them. One day he kissed his new girl friend and a few minutes later his lips blew up like sausages, pink and tender. An hour earlier his girl friend had been eating fish and chips.

Although he had been prepared to put up with his allergy as long as it only meant keeping himself away from fish, he felt it was asking rather a lot to make his girl friend give up her favourite meal too.

The standard way of handling anaphylaxis is to give a shot of adrenalin or epinephrine, which immediately increases blood-pressure and relaxes the air passages. Anaphylactic reactions are fortunately rare: they most often strike people who are highly sensitive to bee and wasp stings, though allergies to foods — particularly fish, buckwheat and egg — are sometimes to blame. Dr Frankland had one American girl patient who had to carry adrenalin with her wherever she went because she was acutely allergic to nuts. If she passed a food counter displaying nuts, she would wheeze. She had almost died on her honeymoon after eating an ice cream which, unbeknown to her, had nuts in it.

During an anaphylactic attack it can be difficult to give yourself a shot of adrenalin. The drug also loses its strength quite quickly, so the allergic person has to keep buying regular fresh supplies.

These disadvantages encouraged doctors to look for other methods of helping this group of their patients.

The technique Dr Frankland used for food allergy was based on the desensitization therapy his predecessors Noon and Freeman had used at St Mary's for pollen allergy. Patients would be admitted to the hospital and given seven injections of their allergen a day, starting with tiny doses of about a millionth of a gram, and gradually working up to much higher doses. The allergen extracts for fish were made from dried, defatted fish steeped in a solution containing 0.4 phenol, which was then added to a saline extracting fluid. The resulting extract was subsequently diluted to the required strength. Despite the minute doses of antigen they were exposed to in the first few shots some patients would react violently. So beside the bed were kept supplies of adrenalin, oxygen and even a surgeon's tracheotomy set to open the windpipe if all else failed.

The young man with the fish problem was warned that rush desensitization like this was a risky procedure, but he was keen to try it. As cod was the fish he was most likely to encounter, Dr Frankland chose cod for the base of the extract. Allergens frequently 'cross-react' with others in the same biological family, so there was a fair chance that if he was desensitized against cod he might also be protected against other fish.

Sadly this was not to be the case this time. The first evening after being discharged the young man had a celebration cod dinner with his girl friend, and felt fine. The next evening he ate a kipper, and was soon on his way to the emergency department.

Food desensitization seems to be rather like influenza vaccination, though much more hazardous. A flu vaccine can only be really effective if it contains samples of the latest virus to evolve. Last year's virus may give a degree of protection, but is never 100 per cent effective. Similarly Dr Frankland's cod antigen might have helped some patients with general fish allergy, but was only really reliable against cod. The other great disadvantage of rush desensitization is that its effects only last about six weeks to two months without being boosted regularly. As it was not feasible to hospitalize his patients as often as that, Dr Frankland would give some patients doses of extract to inject themselves, especially if they were acutely allergic to very common foods like egg or milk.

Another desensitization technique has been invented by Dr Leonard McEwen, a pharmacologist who joined the staff of the St Mary's allergy clinic about fifteen years ago. It took him some time to realize how common food allergy was and even longer to develop his therapy of 'enzyme potentiated hyposensitization'. Many specialists are still sceptical about this therapy, but the story behind its development may give more insight into the problems of food allergy.

As a young registrar Dr McEwen had been puzzled by a particular type of patient who came to the allergy clinic. They were mostly elderly patients who suffered badly from rhinitis or hay fever, often to such an extent that they had lost their sense of smell and had nasal polyps — small tumour-like growths in their noses. The odd thing about them was that the conventional skin tests used to detect allergens always turned out negative. Unlike most allergic patients, who develop a small weal when a solution containing their allergens is pricked into their skin, they did not appear to react to any of the known allergens.

This sort of condition is generally called 'intrinsic allergy', and because allergists could not find a sure explanation for it, they conventionally put it down to autoimmunity. Autoimmunity could be described as a body's allergy to part of itself. This may sound strange, but in several diseases the immune system mistakes certain healthy body cells for dangerous invading organisms and sets about getting rid of them. No one has found a complete explanation for how this happens, but autoimmunity is believed to play a major part in rheumatoid arthritis, ulcerative colitis and some kinds of anaemia.

Dr McEwen did not really care for this explanation of intrinsic allergy. His mistrust had been sparked off by two observations. Firstly, he had heard from some 'intrinsic' patients that they were sensitive to certain foods. Secondly, some patients had told him that they got better when they happened to be on antibiotics or had been taking Entero-Vioform, the antibacterial drug once used for dysentery.

As there was no good reason why an antibiotic should relieve a supposedly autoimmune disease, he wondered whether it might not be worth looking for another cause. The stomach — and what went into it — seemed a good place to start.

He had already seen plenty of patients who were obviously allergic to various foods. Whenever they took a bite of fish, or strawberry, or egg, or whatever they were allergic to, their lips would immediately swell. If the food passed any further than their lips, their tongue and throat would inflame and swell, and if they were unlucky enough to swallow a mouthful they would be violently sick and get an attack of diarrhoea. These patients suffer from acute, or Type One, allergy, which can pretty safely be attributed to immunological causes. Obviously contact between the allergen and antibodies in the mouth was making the mast cells explode in a riot of histamine. Not only that, but these patients have positive reactions to skin tests for food allergens; and high levels of IgE, the antibody associated with allergy, can invariably be found in their blood and tissues.

The 'intrinsic' patients who had told him that they too were sensitive to certain foods did not react this way. They told him that they only experienced the ill effects several hours or sometimes days after eating or drinking the suspect commodity.

The obvious advice for these people was 'Stay off the foods which give you symptoms'. Dr McEwen also began routinely to suggest to patients that they should look out for foods which might be giving them problems and to see what happened if they avoided them. At the same time he found that mothers of young children with eczema were saying that certain foods appeared to make the rash worse.

As the advice he was giving generally seemed to be having a good effect he decided to put the idea to the test. He devised a series of diets which excluded the foods which most commonly caused allergic reactions. As well as following the diet the patients were to be given a regular dose of 250 mg of Entero-Vioform, three times a day.

For his study Dr McEwen selected forty-seven patients. Most of them were suffering from intrinsic rhinitis or asthma, though he also included a number of children and teenagers with eczema.

For the first three weeks they were asked to follow Diet No. 1:

Not to be eaten

Milk — except *Carnation* evaporated milk
Egg, custard, salad dressing, chicken
Nuts and fruits: i.e., tomatoes, blackcurrants and all berries;
oranges and other citrus fruits; fruit juice and fruit drinks;
marmalade; jam; chocolate; fresh coffee; fruit sweets; melons;
cucumber; marrow; peas; beans; peanuts; nuts; marzipan; spices
and curry; cooking oils (peanut or olive)
Fish
Cheese
Onions
Alcohol
Pork, bacon, all liver
Shellfish
Honey
Chewing gum

You can eat

Carnation brand milk only — ½ pint per day, diluted with water.
Cornflakes and other breakfast cereals, oatmeal, oats, rice,
cornflour
Tea and instant coffee
Sugar
Bread, pastry, cakes, biscuits, avoiding cream cakes and ones
with much egg in them
Butter (in small quantities), corn oil, or lard for cooking
Beef, salt beef, beef sausage, lamb
Green vegetables (but *not* cauliflower), lettuce, carrots,
mushrooms (but not more than ¼ lb per week and not all at once)
Potatoes
Apples, pears, bananas (avoiding the cores — and don't eat too
many)
Rhubarb, pineapple

The first question anyone who reads this diet must ask is 'Why does he forbid milk but allow *Carnation*?' The reason is that *Carnation* is produced by heating milk to 103° centigrade for a few minutes, which results in the destruction of the particular protein which is responsible for most allergic reactions to milk. Other brands of evaporated milk might do as well, but he recommended this particular brand because he knew how it was made.

If you recall the advice given by clinical ecologists earlier in this chapter you may be wondering why Dr McEwen allowed his patients to include wheat products in their diet. He did it simply to make the diet easier to follow; but if after three weeks they felt no better, he gave them the much stricter Diet No. 2:

You may eat only

Sugar
Oatmeal, rice
Beef or minced beef
Green vegetables and lettuce
Potatoes
Butter (in small quantities), lard for cooking
Oat cakes
Water or tea without milk or lemon
Rhubarb

Diet No. 2 avoids not only wheat but also milk and fruit. Sticklers among clinical ecologists might object at this point that he was still including plenty of items which are known to be the source of some people's problems. However, his aim was to keep his patients interested by offering them a diet which they could be reasonably expected to follow. In fact out of his forty-seven patients, only two said they found the regime impossible to follow. A couple more — one a student, the other a seaman — lived institutional lives in which they had little choice in the diet they were offered. A few more simply gave up trying after a few days, and another one or two said they preferred to stick with the drug treatment they had been having before. But out of the original forty-seven he was still left with thirty-five at the end of two months who were happy to continue to the next stage.

Diet No. 3 was designed to identify the foods which might be causing problems. The instructions they were given to take home with them ran thus:

Now you have found that your allergy is helped by dieting, you can start again on each group of foods you have left out to see which ones give you trouble. To be sure, you must not start on more than one group of food per week, and you should eat a lot so it will be obvious if it is one of these groups to which you are allergic. The best scheme is:

Week
1. Milk — at least a pint a day
2. Eggs and chicken
3. Nuts and fruits: plenty of tomatoes, some nuts (almonds and brazils, preferably), peas, etc.
4. Fish
5. Cheese
6. Onions and garlic
7. Pork

Whenever you find a food which upsets you, you must go back to the old diet and wait till you are free of symptoms before going on to try a new food.

Foods which do not upset you may be added into your diet after you have tried them out for a week.

If you found the second diet was better for you, then you must also try yourself with wheat products — bread, biscuits, etc., in the first week, and start with milk in the second week.

It therefore took everyone another two months to finish the whole course of the diet. But for the majority of them it proved a very worthwhile exercise. Of the thirty-five patients, only five were no better. Dr McEwen did not make his own judgement about how the remainder had fared, but arranged for them to be assessed at their final visit by his chief, Dr Frankland. Overall, five of them were found to be completely relieved of their symptoms, while another eighteen were 'three-quarters better' and a further seven 'half better'.

Of course the diet was only part of the treatment they had been taking. Throughout the three months of the trial they had also been prescribed Entero-Vioform. At the time this was a very popular medicine, which many people used to take with them on long trips in case they got an attack of stomach troubles abroad. It is much less popular today because it is known to cause temporary damage to nerves if taken for prolonged periods, and it can give some people a hypersensitivity to iodine, a trace element in water and food, which leads to depression, insomnia or sexual impotence. The hazards of prolonged use of Entero-Vioform only began to come to light after Dr McEwen had started his trial, and this naturally put him in a quandary.

Rather than call off the whole trial and thereby lose the chance of putting what appeared to be a useful treatment to the test, he decided to press on; but he warned his patients to look out for any apparent side-effects. In fact three of them did complain after a few weeks of a slight numbness in their hands and feet, but when they were taken off the Entero-Vioform this quickly cleared up.

At the end of the three-month course all the patients were taken off the drug, but they were asked to continue with their new diets and to avoid the foods which they now knew to be responsible for causing their symptoms. At this stage it emerged that several of them needed the Entero-Vioform as much as the diet, because during the next four weeks ten of them relapsed. Although twenty-five of the thirty-five continued happily on their diets without the drug, the others got back their symptoms until they were given another prescription of Entero-Vioform. Indeed, three of those ten only seemed to benefit from the drug; the diet appeared to contribute nothing to their improvement.

Although the drug was obviously helping some patients, Dr McEwen was puzzled as to *why* it should be helping them. Apparently it was having some kind of effect on the bacteria in their stomach and intestines, but exactly what that effect was he was never able to determine.

Apart from this puzzling phenomenon, what were the important chacteristics of his patients' food allergies? Unlike the Type One food-allergic person, who would react immediately and sometimes violently to an allergic food, these people had very delayed reactions. For instance, while they were on Diet No. 3 and gradually reintroducing themselves to the foods they had been avoiding, most patients took more than a day to develop a reaction to a particular food which proved to be allergenic. Only one patient got a reaction within two hours, and only three others reacted within twelve hours. For the majority it took longer than twenty-four hours before they got an attack of asthma, eczema or rhinitis, and a few did not feel the adverse effects of their food till four days later.

It had taken considerably longer for their symptoms to disappear in the first place. On Diet No. 1 it took most of them at least ten days and sometimes as long as three weeks for their symptoms to clear. Response to Diet No. 2 tended to be quicker; all wheat-sensitive patients got better within a week.

The other interesting finding was that nearly everybody turned out to be sensitive to more than one food. Out of thirty cases, only one patient was sensitive to a single food. Five were sensitive to two foods; five to three foods; five to four foods; two to five foods; four to six foods; and three were sensitive to seven of the groups of foods Dr McEwen had identified.

By far and away the most culpable group of foods were the fruits, berries and nuts. Three quarters of his patients had adverse reactions when they ate some kind of food in this group. Over half of them reacted to milk and/or cheese and/or egg. Next in line were pork, yeast-based foods, fish, onions and wheat.

Interestingly, many of his patients told him that they had a particular liking for the foods which were doing them harm and had often devoured them in large amounts.

The best way for these people to get better was to give up the offending foods. But for some, especially those who had to eat in restaurants and canteens, this was not at all easy. So McEwen wondered if there was another way of helping them.

The man who set him on the trail of fresh possibilities was Dr Popper, an ear, nose and throat surgeon from Czechoslovakia. Dr Popper had been an eminent member of his profession before the Second World War. But he was Jewish, and when the Nazis invaded his homeland he fled to Britain. Despite his long professional experience as a surgeon, his qualifications were not recognized by the General Medical Council, the body which grants doctors their licence to practise in Britain. To have been allowed to work as a surgeon he would have had to take the Fellowship exam of the Royal College of Surgeons. As far as practical skills were concerned he was certainly knowledgeable enough to pass with distinction; but a large part of that exam is written, and Dr Popper's English was not really up to the mark. He was also well into middle age and did not have a great inclination to spend a few years boning up on the basics. But although he was not allowed to operate on patients surgically, he was granted a licence to practise as a physician. There were enough of his compatriots in Britain for him to establish a small private practice in Harley Street. And in the course of time he managed to secure part-time work, albeit rather humble for a man of his previous status, in a hospital in Hackney.

Many of the patients who consulted him were afflicted with nasal polyps, the tumour-like growths which grow in the noses of people who have had allergic asthma for many years. These polyps are not malignant tumours; they are in fact little bags containing a jellified substance, hyaluronic acid. Dr Popper reasoned that a simple way to get rid of polyps might be to inject them with hyaluronidase, an enzyme which is extracted from rams' testicles, and which — as its name implies — breaks down hyaluronic acid.

He duly set about injecting the polyps of about thirty patients, but with little success. He would have abandoned the therapy there and then but for the fact that his patients started returning to him a few weeks or months later to tell him that the sneezing fits and runny noses they used to get when exposed to pollen had disappeared. Although he could not think why this should be, he persevered with the injections, and found that a signficant number of his patients benefited this way, and that the effect could last for up to two years after their injection.

Realizing that he had probably stumbled on a very useful new treatment for allergy, he approached a leading drug company, Bencard, and asked them to support his investigations. Keen to exploit what might prove to be a breakthrough, the drug company provided Dr Popper with preparations of hyaluronidase and encouraged him to keep up the good work. Unfortunately the results he got from Bencard's hyaluronidase were disappointing. It was not so much that the treatment no longer worked, but rather that it worked for some groups of patients and not others. His two previous years of success had convinced him that it should work, so he carried on. After another year he realized what the problem was: some batches of hyaluronidase were effective, but others were not.

Unwillling to accept that their preparations were faulty, Bencard decided to stop sponsoring Dr Popper's work. Annoyed but not yet defeated, Dr Popper persuaded a small drug company, Biorex, to help him continue. By now it was the mid-1960s, and Dr McEwen was already working at St Mary's Hospital. The allergy department at St Mary's was asked by Biorex whether they would help with the project, and Dr McEwen was given the task of assessing the patients Dr Popper was treating.

Biorex went to great lengths to produce supplies of hyaluronidase which were as pure as possible. Confident that the treatment would work, they invested £20,000 (a considerable sum twenty years ago) in the project and arranged that a total of eight allergists around the country would try hyaluronidase on their patients. Sadly the project failed to produce any useful results. The doctors found that the Biorex preparation appeared to work no better than a placebo injection of salt solution. Aggrieved to see their investment in expensive rams' testicles so sadly squandered, the company abrupty withdrew their sponsorship of Dr Popper's research. This discouragement was perhaps the last straw for the lonely émigré; within a year he had had two coronaries and had died.

Dr McEwen did not share the drug company's view. Won over by poor Dr Popper's enthusiam he decided to take the investigation further. Before long he found that he was having the same experience with the enzyme preparations as Dr Popper had had in the early work sponsored by Bencard. Certain batches worked, but others did not.

Now these preparations are notoriously difficult to purify, and Dr McEwen wondered whether it was the hyaluronidase which had been making patients better or whether it might not be something else in the injections, something which might previously have been regarded as a contaminant, which was making the therapy work. So he went to the company which was making his hyaluronidase and asked its chemists to tell him frankly what the known contaminants of the preparations were. They told him that there were in fact several enzymes which were difficult to separate from hyaluronidase. The most significant one was called beta-glucuronidase.

To test his hunch Dr McEwen embarked on a series of experiments which were to last several years. In his first tests guinea pigs and mice were sensitized to various allergens, and then attempts were made to desensitize them by using beta-glucuronidase or hyaluronidase with small quantities of the antigen. In some experiments the enzymes were used singly with the antigen, sometimes they were combined, sometimes they were combined with other enzymes which were thought to have some possible role in the way the therapy worked. After several years of experimentation he worked out a recipe which did produce consistently good results.

The recipe Dr McEwen uses today contains both beta-glucuronidase and hyaluronidase, together with two other substances, protamine and cyclohexane. They are put together into a solution with extracts of a variety of foods. When a patient comes to be desensitized, the doctor scrapes off an area of skin on the forearm about a quarter of an inch square with a blunt lancet. He uses a blunt edge because a sharp blade is likely to nick the skin and draw blood. The aim is to let the solution slowly percolate through the skin, so after the top, waterproof layer of skin has been removed, a small thimble-shaped plastic cup which holds 1 cc of the solution is strapped over the area and left in place for a day. By 1979 about 4,000 patients had been treated in this way. They come back for a top-up desensitization every three or four months. Certainly the technique does not cure everyone, but Dr McEwen claims that the majority of patients are able to eat freely of the foods which previously caused them trouble.

The great virtues of this hyposensitization treatment are its safety and cheapness. Although it sounds very complicated to prepare, each three-monthly dose costs only a few pennies to produce.

Nevertheless it is not widely used. The main reason for this is that few British doctors are interested in food allergy and have therefore not had any inclination to try it. Also, despite its apparent success in Dr McEwen's hands, it has not yet been tested by a double-blind trial, and is therefore regarded as unproven.

If it does work, we are still left with the question *how*. Many allergists believe that all desensitization methods work by stimulating the immune system to produce a protective antibody, IgA. IgA does not attach itself to mast cells like IgE and therefore does not spark off inflammation. It also seems to act as a first line of defence, intercepting antigens before they activate the white blood cells which produce IgA. Although Dr McEwen has found no evidence that his technique boosts IgA, it does seem that the protective agent, whatever it may be, is circulating in the bloodstream. His animal experiments have shown that immunity to an allergen can be passed on by injecting an animal with blood taken from another which has been desensitized by his method. He has also noticed that if a desensitized patient loses a lot of blood, the previous sensitivity returns.

The role of the protamine and cyclohexane is also something of a mystery, even to him. They are included because they potentiate, or activate, the enzymes. During the course of his experiments Dr McEwen found that these substances had a remarkable effect. In large quantities (and when I say large, I am talking about thousandths of a gram!) they increase the desensitizing effect, but if the quantity is reduced a hundredfold they do the opposite — they make the patient hypersensitive. Going down one stage further they desensitized, but if taken one stage further the effect was reversed yet again. This strange phenomenon is reminiscent of the sublingual switch-on/switch-off effect and of the way pollen-sensitive patients can react to large and minute doses of pollen in a prick test.

More Ways of Diagnosing Food and Chemical Allergy

The only sure way of testing yourself for food or chemical allergy is to avoid the suspect substance for a long time and to see whether that makes you feel better. To clinch the diagnosis you then have to be exposed to the substance again and see whether your symptoms return. As many foods are very difficult and some chemicals nigh impossible to avoid, this is a counsel of perfection.

There are two laboratory tests which aid diagnosis. The newest is the unpronounceable *radioallergosorbent test*, usually simply known as RAST. Without going into technicalities, RAST determines whether body fluids or tissues contain antibodies which react specifically to a suspended allergen. The main drawback of RAST is that even if it shows that antibodies are present, there is no certainty that the patient is allergic to that substance. We develop antibodies to many foreign proteins to which we are often exposed, but we do not always become sensitized to them. However, RAST is much more reliable than skin tests for diagnosing food allergy.

Cytotoxic tests reveal whether foods or chemicals are harming white blood cells. Samples of blood are taken and added to a weak solution of the food or chemical. If cells have been sensitized to an antigen, they will be destroyed more quickly than normal cells. This process is observed through a microscope, and the degree of sensitivity is estimated by counting the cells remaining after about three quarters of an hour.

The advantage of cytotoxic tests is that one sample of blood from the patient will give the laboratory technician enough blood cells to test reactions to many possible allergens. They are therefore very useful for diagnosing multiple allergies, which are in fact more common than allergies to a single food. Reactions can also be tested to chemicals which would prove dangerous or highly unpleasant if administered directly to the patient. Cytotoxic tests may not reveal every allergy, because they cannot tell us anything about reactions to food which occur after the food has been broken down in the stomach. It seems likely that some food allergies are the result of reactions to proteins which have been partially transformed during digestion and which bear little similarity to their original form.

Many food allergists believe that a masked allergy can lead to a serious depletion of white cells. As white cells are the principal forces of the immune system, a depletion can make the body vulnerable to attack from other invaders such as bacteria and viruses. Dr Ted Randolph has found, and others have confirmed, that if a patient eats a food to which he or she is allergic, the white blood cell population drops and remains lower than normal for as long as the food continues to be eaten. It returns to normal if the food is cut out of the diet. Obviously if someone is just mildly intolerant to many foods, the accumulative effect on the white cell population will prove to be as bad as exposure to a single very potent poison. For this reason clinical ecologists may warn their patients against common foods even if the cytotoxic test suggests that these foods are only mildly toxic. This practice has provoked an accusation that the ecologists are alarming their patients unnecessarily. The ecologists reply that there is no need for alarm, because food allergy is not always permanent; if a food is given up for a while and then reintroduced slowly and in small amounts, the patient may come to tolerate it. This can only happen when the worst food and chemical allergens have been eliminated and the body's defences have had a chance to get back on an even keel.

Generally speaking, though, the cytotoxic test must be treated with a lot of caution. One laboratory which offers the test — for fees of up to £120 — has recently been shown up by investigations by *The Observer* newspaper and the Channel 4 health programme *Well Being*. People who were known to have very strong allergies to particular foods sent in their blood samples but were diagnosed as having allergies quite different from their actual ones. Healthy people without any known allergies at all were told they had a whole range of food allergies.

Of the various alternative medical approaches to allergy perhaps the strangest diagnostic technique is *radionic analysis*. A pendulum is swung over a sample of hair or blood from the patient — who need not be on the scene at all — and the practitioner judges from the direction in which it swings whether or not the patient has an allergy to the substance. This technique is said to be related to water divining, but — from my experience — it seems to be even less reliable. Like the cytotoxic test it completely missed some very strong allergies and diagnosed some very unlikely ones.

Diagnosis by diet

In time laboratory tests may become more accurate and useful, but they cannot yet replace diets as the most reliable guide to diagnosis. Earlier in this chapter, I described one kind of elimination diet used by Dr McEwen, which was derived from the diets successfully pioneered by Dr Rowe many years before. I shall give some more detailed diets later on, but first I would like to mention the basic methods.

Of course we do not usually call for a diagnosis unless we have something to complain about. So let's begin by going through diseases which have been attributed to food and chemical allergy. (Of course it must be emphasized that allergy is not necessarily the only cause of these complaints.)

Respiratory complaints: asthma (wheezing); rhinitis (runny and/or itchy nose); bronchitis. These are often accompanied by conjunctivitis (red, runny eyes).

Stomach, gut and bladder: colic; colitis; diarrhoea; ulcers; bed-wetting; gallstones; vomiting.

Skin: eczema; mouth ulcers; rashes and hives; persistent itches and soreness.

Muscles and joints: arthritis; aches and pains with no obvious cause.

Heart and circulation: racing pulse; spasms and pains which resemble angina or heart attacks; high blood-pressure; inexplicable blanching, blushing or fainting; migraine.

Mind, emotions and nervous system: depression; schizophrenia; mania (elation or aggression alternating irrationally with lethargy); panic attacks; inability to concentrate; hyperactivity (especially in children); convulsions and fits; numbness in various parts; vertigo; ringing in the ears.

Cancer has been attributed to food allergy. Prolonged exposure to an irritant or severe pressure on the immune system can impair the body's ability to check malignant cells. Allergy to the various ingredients of cigaretttes could explain why some heavy smokers get lung cancer while others (in fact the majority) do not.

Heart disease and hardening of the arteries are associated with fatty diets, though we still do not know why all people who eat the same diet do not seem to suffer in the same way.

Food and chemical allergy may not be the only cause or even

the most common cause of these diseases, but it is almost certainly the most unrecognized cause. I am of course using the term 'allergy' in its widest meaning; only a minority of the complaints listed fit the orthodox description of allergy. It may turn out that antibodies and immunological mechanisms do play a part in many of these diseases, but for our present purposes that is not important. Allergy here means intolerance.

It seems that any food can produce almost any symptom in someone who is allergic to it. Some authors of books and articles on food allergy associate certain foods with certain symptoms, but no opinion ever seems to concur exactly with another. Dr McEwen has found that among his wheat-sensitive patients he has some who get rhinitis, some who get nasal polyps, some who get eczema, some who get migraine, some who get itchy eyes, some who get stomach troubles, some who get aches and pains in muscles and joints, some who get epileptic fits and others who suffer mentally.

Antigen/antibody reactions are only part of the picture. Many people who suffer from migraine, for instance, get their attacks after eating foods which are rich in a substance called tyramine. Chocolate, pickled herrings, broad beans, cheese and red wine are the most notorious in this respect. For most of us tyramine presents no problems, because we have enzymes which break it down quickly; but some migraineurs seem to lack these enzymes. If tyramine builds up in the blood, it provokes a series of reactions which leads to constriction of blood vessels in the head, which causes the pain. An immunologist would therefore say that migraine was not an allergy, because it was not caused by an abnormal immune reaction. In the wide, popular sense of the word, however, migraine can be the result of an allergy, i.e. intolerance of tyramine-rich foods.

You might think that the easiest way to diagnose food allergy would be to feed yourself large quantities of a suspect food and see if it made you ill. This would work if you had an acute allergy, but it would then be both unnecessary and hazardous. We have also seen that many allergies are to favourite foods. In this case reactions are delayed and may be masked by a lift we get whenever we eat the food again. As in the case of Dr Rinkel, who first tried to diagnose his egg allergy by swallowing six raw eggs at once, excessive feeding does not disclose this kind of addiction.

The best way to identify a masked allergy or addiction is to give the food up for about five days and then eat it. As Dr Rinkel discovered when he ate the angel food cake, the effect can be shattering, but it is not always so bad. If symptoms do not clear up during the five days of abstinence, it may be worth persevering for up to two weeks before testing yourself. If the symptoms do clear up, the food may be their cause, but you still have to challenge yourself with a generous quantity of the food and watch for the symptoms to return — perhaps a few days later — before you can be reasonably certain. Even then, you should not be too dogmatic. Food may be an important factor, but it is not necessarily the only cause of the symptoms. Indeed, it would be unwise to embark upon a dietary diagnosis without medical supervision or at least without having ensured that any severe symptoms do not have some other treatable cause.

If exclusion of one food makes no difference to your condition, it is probably — but not necessarily — safe. It is common to be allergic to more than one food, in which case your symptoms are unlikely to disappear unless you eliminate all the allergens.

As eggs, milk, wheat, corn and chemicals in foods and packaging are the most common allergens the next stage might be to exclude all these things. Eggs, milk and flour are universal in processed foods, so nothing but fresh foods should be eaten. If you feel better after following this diet you can begin to add the excluded foods back into it one by one, leaving three days between each, to see whether they provoke a reaction.

Food diaries are recommended by some clinical ecologists. Over a period of weeks you take note of everything you eat at each meal every day and also take note of any symptoms you experience. Food diaries are useful for picking out the more unusual allergenic foods, but generally they are rather cumbersome. Delayed reactions may make you suspect innocent foods. If you eat out in a restaurant, you will probably not know exactly what you have eaten anyway. Doctors who get their patients to keep food diaries often eventually realize that the diary is forgotten until the day before the patient's next appointment: to keep the doctor happy the patient is tempted to cobble together an account which probably omits vital details.

Food diaries are more useful if they are combined with a strict elimination diet. An elimination diet begins by restricting you to foods which are only rarely associated with allergy: lamb, pears, rice, rye, green vegetables and olive oil might be a basic diet of this kind. This diet is kept up for a week to allow all traces of the old diet to pass out of the system, and then more suspect foods are added, one by one, and in generous quantities. If an adverse reaction occurs, the new food is discarded again and you revert to the safe foods until your symptoms disappear before proceeding further.

As symptoms may take a few days to show up, new foods should not be added too quickly. According to Dr J. C. Breneman, Chairman of the American College of Allergists' Food Allergy Committee and author of the medical textbook *Basics of Food Allergy*, symptoms appear in a quite predictable and typical way:

Heartburn and indigestion within half an hour of eating the offending food.

Headache usually within one hour.

Rhinitis and asthma in one hour.

Bloating stomach and diarrhoea within three or four hours.

Hives and rashes within six to twelve hours.

A noticeable gain in weight caused by water retention in twelve to fifteen hours.

Fits, confusion 'and other mental aberrations' within twelve to twenty-four hours.

Aphthous (mouth) ulcers, aching joints, muscles or back in forty-eight to ninety-six hours.

Some might dispute whether this timetable was 100 per cent reliable, but it conforms generally with the observations of doctors I have met. Note that these reactions take much longer than those provoked by sublingual tests, which follow within minutes or seconds. The difference is that sublingual drops are readily absorbed into the blood-stream and reach their target more quickly.

The basic 'cleansing' diet should be recommended for all patients with confusing symptoms or unexplained disabilities, Dr Breneman declares: 'The response may be so rewarding that both physician and patient ask: "Why didn't we do this sooner?"'

The order he suggests for introducing new foods is as follows:

milk, beef, wheat, egg, corn, chicken, orange, potato, pork. Each is eaten regularly for three days before you go onto the next. The foods just listed are the most common allergens. Once they have been tested you move on to coffee, beans, nuts, citrus fruits, shellfish and other types of food, devoting three days to each new addition. The investigation is rounded off with tests of food preservatives and common medicines. Aspirin and antibiotics turn out to be quite frequent allergens.

Anyone who is sensitive to aspirin may also react badly to the food colouring tartrazine or to any of the many natural foods which contain salicylates. These include almonds, apples, apricots, several berry fruits, strawberries, raisins and wines. Salicylates are also often found in cosmetics, mouthwashes, toothpastes, chewing gum and soft drinks. (A more detailed list is given in Appendix IV at the back of this book.)

Groups of foods may turn out to be as allergenic as individual foods. Some people who are allergic to tomatoes, for instance, are allergic to other members of the same plant family, which includes green peppers, aubergines, tobacco and potatoes. (Lists of the most important food families are also given in the back of this book in Appendix III.)

According to Dr Len McEwen, allergies to many or all the foods in the fruit and nut group are common. He claims that he can desensitize people who are allergic to, say, apples or oranges by giving them an extract of mixed nuts which does not contain the fruit that actually brings on their symptoms. He suggests that there may be a common allergen in all fruits and nuts which is probably found in the seed. He points out that most of his patients who are allergic to fruit can avoid an adverse reaction if they are careful not to eat the seeds or the pith. One girl only reacted to oranges if she ate the seeds or if she ate home-made marmalade. Marmalade caused problems because her mother followed the traditional recipe, which involves suspending a muslin bag of orange seeds in the saucepan.

Elimination diets barely touch on the possible chemical and airborne allergens in the environment. Pollen, spores, dust mites and animal danders have long been recognized as the causes of asthma. Respiratory complaints are only mild afflictions compared with some of the ills wafted to us on the breeze. Moulds, the minute fungi which proliferate particularly well in damp environments, have been blamed for a wide range of mental symptoms. The American allergist Dr Marshall Mandell has filmed the reactions of patients to sublingual drops containing mould extracts: as well as provoking mild mental distress in the form of anxiety, vertigo, headaches and anger, the moulds made some patients acutely depressed while others burst into tears, and one woman went catatonic for three quarters of an hour.

Moulds are also responsible for farmer's lung and the various occupational diseases mentioned earlier. Penicillin is made from a mould. Although this kind of mould has proved very useful in medicine, we should not forget that its power comes from its ability to release a toxin which kills bacteria. The antibiotic streptomycin has been known to cause severe damage to cranial nerves, and several of the antibiotics derived from related fungi have similar dangers. Antibiotics are well known for their ability to cause rashes, breathing problems and other allergic complaints; many thousands of people have to carry cards or bracelets warning doctors not to give them penicillin or similar antibiotics if they are admitted to a hospital.

Ergot, a mould which grows on rye, contains some alkaloids which have medicinal uses and others which are related chemically to LSD and cause hallucinations. In the Middle Ages whole European communities were reguarly stricken with Saint Anthony's fire, a disease caused by eating flour made from mouldy rye, which led to convulsions. Aflatoxins, one of the most potent carcinogens, come from moulds which grow on peanuts and soya beans.

Perhaps not every mould has such acutely toxic properties. Nevertheless there are thousands of kinds of moulds which flourish in homes and workplaces and it would be rash to dismiss them altogether. As moulds like dampness, their favourite breeding places in the home are bathrooms, basements, kitchens, air-conditioning systems and old wallpaper. Damp clothes and the interior of motor cars are also popular terrain. Many asthmatics have been relieved when a source of mould in their home has been identified and eliminated. Perhaps many 'neuroses' and more severe psychiatric problems would respond equally well.

Pneumonitis, an inflammation of the lungs, is often the result of allergy to spores of moulds which flourish in air-conditioning systems. Long before lung damage is visible on X-ray photographs, the sufferer will have a runny, itchy nose, which gradually develops into recurrent feverishness accompanied by tiredness and a loss in weight.

The hydrocarbon chemicals derived from oil and coal are the commonest artificial allergens. As I mentioned earlier, Dr Ted Randolph persuaded many of his patients in Chicago to throw out their gas cookers when they were found to be the cause of headaches and nausea. Exhaust fumes from car engines also affect some people very badly, and are probably the major cause of car sickness. These fumes are not necessarily very smelly or obvious, as this case history shows:

A thirty-six-year-old housewife began to have nausea whenever she went out in the family car. A qualified mechanic examined the exhaust system twice but failed to find any link. But when it was examined a third time with the engine well warmed up, a small crack was noticed on the underside of one of the exhaust manifolds, which closed up when the engine cooled down. When the faulty manifold was replaced the woman's symptoms disappeared.

Phenol is a common ingredient of many domestic products. It is used in plastics, food can linings, drugs, aerosols and disinfectants, to mention a few. It is the cause of many supposedly psychosomatic ailments. Dr Larry Dickey, a senior American clinical ecologist, gave me an example:

One of his female patients first came to him for help with her migraine. All the medicines used for treating migraine had not only failed on her, but had actually made her worse. Her previous doctor had concluded that her migraine was not typical and had referred her to a psychiatrist. She was reluctant to believe that she was mentally ill, even mildly so. A cytotoxic test indicated phenol sensitivity, but in the course of her dietary program she had a migraine after drinking canned tomato juice, which made her think that she must be allergic to tomatoes. But when she drank tomato juice which she had prepared herself from fresh tomatoes and stored in glass bottles, she did not get a migraine. She subsequently found that canned salmon gave her a headache but that bottled salmon did not. In fact whenever she ate food which came from a can lined with phenolic resin she always got a migraine. Phenol had also been used in the manufacture of the drugs which had made her condition worse.

PVC and other plastic fabrics used in furniture and car upholstery contain gases which are slowly released long after manufacture. These can produce a wide range of symptoms in sensitive people. This problem has become more noticeable now that safety laws and car design fashions insist on more protective padding inside cars. Unfortunately, opting for leather upholstery does not necessarily avoid this hazard, as a few people have been found to be sensitive to the tanning chemicals in leather.

Francis Silver, an engineer from West Virginia who has made a specialty of designing safe homes for chemically sensitive people, reports that mattresses and bedding materials are one of the commonest causes of insomnia, lethargy and rashes. The main culprit here seems to be flame retardants, which are almost universally used in bedding to prevent it catching fire, and urethane foam, which gives off gas. The best way of dealing with this problem if you cannot replace your mattress with something more suitable is to cover it with aluminium foil or with an aluminized mattress cover. Sadly, however, aluminium is not problem-free. It can cause skin rashes, and aluminium cooking pots can impart enough metal into boiled foods to make sensitive people quite ill. Aluminium poisoning could therefore easily be confused with food allergy.

Most homes contain a mass of paints, sprays, disinfectants and sundry chemical liquids which have been accumulated over the years and left forgotten in cupboards and basements. Francis Silver tells of one of his clients who complained of itching, burning and a crawling feeling on her skin:

Dustbins full of cans and bottles were removed from the house and put outside in the yard. A can of *Roost-no-more* bird-repellent was found on a shelf under the stairs. The protective cap was missing, and another shelf rested on a spray button, so whenever anyone walked down the stairs the shelves bounced up and down and delivered a small squirt of *Roost-no-more* into the air with each bounce. This was probably the worst insult to this woman's skin of a huge number of possible sources.

Silver cites another case, where the chemical allergen was less obvious:

A woman who had become very chemical-sensitive found that she could not leave her bedroom and go anywhere else in the house without discomfort. She could not even stay in her bathroom more than a few seconds. About a bushel of various cans and bottles were removed from the bathroom. In several weeks she was comfortable in her bathroom for longer periods, though exactly what had been the cause of her trouble was not identified. Probably no one thing was responsible but rather the sum of tiny contributions from many different sources. Several barrels were removed from the remainder of the house and in a few years she could go comfortably throughout the building except in the basement, where chlordane insecticide had been used.

Now, when I showed this case report to a doctor who was rather sceptical about the alleged hazards of chemicals, he delared that there was no hard evidence here to prove that the chemicals were to blame.

'I think this woman could simply have been so alarmed by the ecologists' propaganda that she got a neurosis about chemicals and imagined them everywhere doing her harm,' he suggested.

This is the opinion with which many orthodox practitioners would concur. But it brings us no nearer to understanding why the lady was likely to become 'neurotic' in the first place. The majority of patients who consult family doctors today are women (they outnumber men in a ratio of sixty to forty), and their most frequent complaints are mild anxieties, depression, inability to cope with other mental upsets. These ailments make very big business for the manufacturers of tranquillizers, but they are seldom really cured. When we consider that housewives spend the greater part of their time in the same house exposed consistently to the same chemical pollutants, is it not conceivable that chemical allergy could be the cause of their problems?

Alarming people is not necessarily a bad thing in this context. Most of us are frankly unaware of what goes into our modern environment. Technology is held in general awe, and most people take it on trust that their air, water, food and domestic materials are safe. Sadly, our trust has shaky foundations.

I have only given the barest outline of the known hazards of the invisible chemical environment. The best way to make a sure diagnosis of chemical allergy is to see how you respond to an environment free of suspected allergens. Clinical ecologists use sublingual drops containing chemicals to provoke symptoms and to switch them off. Phenol and ethanol in very dilute form are used for diagnosing and treating a wide range of chemical problems, and anyone who is very sensitive to any chemical is likely to react to phenol and/or ethanol drops. Clinical ecologists are very careful about finding out about the source of their test samples. Ethanol can be made by fermenting sugar or by refining oil; although a chemist would say that they were identical, clinical ecologists claim that these ethanols are quite distinct and retain the allergic potential of the substance from which they are derived.

The most exhaustive and comprehensive method for diagnosing food and chemical allergy is the environmental unit. Pioneered by Dr Ted Randolph in Chicago and Dr William Rea in Dallas, Texas, environmental units are designed to take you right away from all the possible chemical allergens which are impossible to avoid at home. The units are situated in rural or suburban areas where there is minimal atmospheric pollution, and every possible attempt is made to ensure that the air inside the unit is uncontaminated. Incoming air has to be passed through carbon filters. Electrical or hot-water heating systems are preferred to gas-fired or warm-air systems, which could spread fumes. Electric fans, however, are banned because of the risk from droplets of oil thrown out by their centrifugal force, and television sets are frowned upon because their plastic components give off fumes when the set is hot. Floors, ideally made of terrazzo tiles, are cleaned with a minimum of disinfectant, and then only with unscented brands. Unscented soap is allowed, but toothpastes, aerosol sprays, perfumes, newspapers and magazines are not permitted. Furnishings are made of cotton, leather and other natural materials, and anything containing feathers, plastic foam, rubber, fireproofing chemicals or plasticized surfaces is eschewed. Pine wood is admitted only if it is well seasoned and preferably varnished — though the varnish should be at least two years old to ensure that it is not still releasing fumes. Any room which is newly painted is left unused until the paint is thoroughly hard and dry and has lost its characteristic fresh smell. Patients are asked to wear only clothes made of natural materials which have never caused them problems. Smokers are told to drop their habit immmediately — but are given the consoling advice that the starvation diet they are about to embark on will probably reduce their craving for cigarettes.

The regime for patients varies slightly according to the doctor, though the usual practice is to begin with a complete fast for five days, drinking only pure spring water and taking a little sea salt. This spartan style may be hard to take at first, and most people feel sharp hunger pangs especially in the first two days, which are sometimes accompanied by a foul taste in the mouth, perspiration, aching and shivers. But Dr Randolph reports that these reactions quickly wear off, and that most patients come through these five days feeling a good deal better than when they started. Foods are then introduced one by one. Those which are particularly suspect are given to the patient firstly in unadulterated form, i.e., organically grown without pesticides or preservatives. If the patient does not react to these pure foods, canned or other commercial forms of the food are then given. This helps to distinguish real food allergy from allergy to chemicals in foods. Once established on a diet they can tolerate, patients will be exposed to common chemicals. Reactions to water are also tested: after spring water, patients are given tap water, artesian well water and a variety of bottled waters to drink. Fluorine and chlorine have been blamed for causing hives, among other things, so water treated with these chemicals is tested too.

This kind of programme is about as rigorous as you can get, but if you are chemically sensitive it is really only the beginning. After you are discharged from the unit you have to return to your normal environment and find out whether, when and in what circumstances your old symptoms come back.

As hospital costs are so high in the United States, the environmental unit is often only used as a last resort. The sceptical attitude of medical insurance corporations towards ecological medicine has discouraged interested parties from setting up more of them. Doctors who run such units find that insurers claim that the two-week stay in an environmental unit is no more than 'a diagnostic procedure' and they refuse to pay the full cost of the stay. These squabbles do not occur in Britain because there are no units like this in the country.

5

Drugs for Allergy

An Aspirin A Day Keeps the Allergy Away?

Whenever aspirin has appeared in this book so far, it has been in the role of 'bad guy'. I have mentioned how some people are acutely sensitive to this drug, and get asthma attacks or break out in a rash whenever they take it. They may also react badly to foods containing salicylates, the chemical family to which aspirin belongs. Aspirin also irritates the stomach wall and causes internal bleeding if it is taken regularly in substantial doses. It would therefore seem reasonable to assume that aspirin is a drug allergic people would do well to avoid.

Strangely though, the reverse appears to be true for some people. While aspirin has for decades been the most widely prescribed and self-prescribed medicine, its workings have only recently begun to be understood. And even now our knowledge is peppered with paradoxes. For instance, about one person in five who suffers from 'intrinsic' asthma (the kind which affects adults rather than children and which often shows up as a delayed reaction to allergenic foods) is sensitive to aspirin. But if you give aspirin to a young person with acute asthma, who has immediate IgE-type reactions to pollen, there is a good chance he will actually do well on it. Recent research has shown that people who are acutely allergic to foods can protect themselves by taking a hefty dose of aspirin before eating.

Before considering how useful aspirin may be in the treatment of food allergy, we must take a brief look at how the drug works. Aspirin and a number of more modern but related drugs such as indomethacin and ibuprofen interfere with the ways the body produces prostaglandins. Prostaglandins are fatty acids generated in almost all body tissues, and their main known function is to constrict and dilate blood vessels and to stimulate smooth muscle — that is, the muscle in internal organs over which we have no apparent control. Prostaglandins are found in the fluids around inflamed tissues, and if you inject prostaglandins into the skin they will cause inflammation.

Prostaglandins are produced by an enzyme breaking down another fatty acid, called arachidonic acid. It is this activity which aspirin and related drugs interfere with. By preventing the enzyme from breaking down arachidonic acid, they check the release of prostaglandins. This in turn impedes inflammation or, in the case of a headache, prevents the excessive dilation or constriction of blood vessels that is usually the cause of the pain.

Although we swallow millions of pills to rid ourselves of the effects of prostaglandins, these substances do have medicinal uses. The stimulatory effect they exert on muscles in the womb, for instance, has made them a useful aid for inducing pregnant women to go into labour, or, if necessary, abort. One of the side-effects of prostaglandin treatment, however, is that it can also cause diarrhoea and vomiting.

Ironically, it was these unwanted side-effects which first suggested that aspirin might be useful for treating food allergy. In 1978 Dr P. D. Buisseret and his colleagues at Guy's Hospital, London, noticed that patients with acute food allergies suffered similar gastrointestinal symptoms to patients who had been prescribed prostaglandins. They wondered whether the allergic reactions might also be caused by prostaglandins, and decided to put this idea to the test.

Let us look at the case histories of some of their patients.

A thirty-eight-year-old woman had been referred to the clinic because she vomited whenever she ate mussels. This problem had been with her for several years, but she noticed that it disappeared after a doctor had prescribed her ibuprofen, an anti-inflammatory drug for her arthritis.

This lady was just the kind of patient Dr Buisseret and his colleagues were interested in, for not only did she have a food allergy, but she also obviously responded well to a drug which stopped prostaglandins. She agreed to help them. They found that if she ate two mussels and then took 400 milligrams of ibuprofen, her symptoms would only be very mild. So far, so good. Unfortunately there was a mix-up at a later stage of the investigation: she was inadvertently allowed to eat six mussels without first receiving the protective drug. Her reaction, as you might expect, was dramatic: within the hour she was prostrate from diarrhoea and vomiting. As she was in no state to swallow anything else, she was given a suppository containing 25 milligrams of indomethacin. Within half an hour she was very much better.

Her rapid response to the anti-inflammatory drug was not the only interesting fact to emerge. They also found that when she ate mussels the prostaglandin levels in her blood rose dramatically, just as the symptoms began to make themselves felt.

Another patient, a thirty-year-old woman, had been suffering from diarrhoea and colicky pains for more than a year. She had lost a lot from weight and felt generally run down and miserable. When she was a teenager she had also suffered a lot from diarrhoea, so badly in fact that she had had a laparotomy, an exploratory operation which allows the surgeon to look for abnormalities in the gut — though in her case nothing obvious had been found. She had been put on an exclusion diet, which had helped her, but she had given it up. Now whenever she ate corn or egg her stomach would puff out within half an hour. Two hours later she would feel sick: diarrhoea would come on after about five hours; and for the next two or three days she would feel out of sorts. These symptoms would sometimes also come on if she consumed bananas, milk products, shellfish, wine or beer. The doctors found that if she was given a 25 milligram tablet of indomethacin before breakfast and then challenged with her 'bad' foods, there would be no sign of her normal symptoms.

Similar findings emerged from their study of several other male and female patients. Prostaglandin levels in the blood would rise about an hour after the allergenic foods had been eaten, but this could be prevented by giving aspirin, indomethacin or ibuprofen. Diarrhoea and vomiting were not the only ills which the drugs could check; some patients had joint pains or runny eyes as well as gut problems and these would also be resolved by the drug treatment. One girl who got a headache and whose eyes streamed whenever she ate tomatoes or drank *Coca-Cola* found that she could escape all harm by taking a couple of aspirin tablets half an hour beforehand.

Aspirin and its pharmacological cousins clearly have a useful role to play in treating food allergy, though there are some big questions still to be resolved. Why does the drug help some allergic people but harm others? This may have something to do with the fact that there are several kinds of prostaglandin, and each has distinct functions. One kind constricts blood vessels, while another dilates them, for instance. Does the aspirin only affect the production of one type of prostaglandin but not the others? Certainly one of the most significant aspects of Dr Buisseret's patients is that there was no obvious immunological explanation for their allergies; they did not have abnormal amounts of antibody to their bad foods. The reactions appeared to be due entirely to some quirk of body chemistry.

I must conclude with a word of warning to anyone who feels tempted to ward off the symptoms of their own food allergy with aspirin. Although it is a very familiar and popular drug, it is not free of hazards. As I pointed out at the beginning of this chapter, it can irritate the gut and is also sometimes a cause of allergic reactions. Like all drugs, it should be treated with caution.

Other Drug Treatments for Allergy

Histamine, like the prostaglandins, is one of the many natural substances which play a part in inflammation. It is released when cells are injured, as, for instance, when an allergen alights on a mast cell coated with IgE antibody. It makes blood vessels dilate, especially the tiny capillary vessels in the skin, which causes redness and heat. By dilating blood vessels it also makes them more permeable, so that plasma, the fluid part of the blood, can seep through the walls of the vessels and thus cause the surrounding tissues to swell. This is the cause of hives, weals and swellings in allergies.

Antihistamine drugs have been used for a long time in the

treatment of hay fever and allergic rashes, though they are not very effective at relieving allergic asthma. Taken before meals they can prevent inflammation in the stomach and gut caused by food allergy. They do not work by stopping injured cells from releasing histamine, but by latching onto the 'receptors' in cells which histamine has to activate to achieve its effect.

Antihistamines unfortunately produce a variety of side-effects which can be as aggravating for the sufferer as the allergic symptoms themselves. The commonest side-effect is drowsiness, which makes them rather unsuitable for people who have to concentrate in their work and daily activities. Although stuffy noses, temporary swellings, insect bites and nettle rash (nettles themselves contain histamine) respond well to antihistamines, there is a danger of actually causing an allergy to the antihistamine itself if the drug is applied too generously to the skin.

Antihistamines are not effective in severe allergic reactions like anaphylaxis. In such cases *adrenalin* is used to open up constricted airways.

Synthetic steroids are man-made forms of hormones. They are highly effective at reducing inflammation, but they have to be given in relatively large doses. If they are administered continuously they encourage the adrenal glands to give up producing natural hormones. As a result a patient who is taken off steroids may suffer an appalling rebound of symptoms since there are no natural reserves left to cope. If on the other hand the patient continues to take steroids, the long-term effects include unusual hairness, 'moon' face, muscle weakness and nervous disorders. Like all strong medicines they offer blessings and curses, and the physician who prescribes steroids has to tread a difficult path. Adrenalin is in fact quicker than steroids at reversing an anaphylaxis.

The drug which has proved most useful for treating food and chemical allergies is *disodium cromoglycate*, better known by its brand names, Intal, Nalcrom and Rynacrom. The drug is believed to work by 'stabilizing' mast cells, thus preventing them from releasing histamine should they be injured in an antigen/antibody reaction. Disodium cromoglycate is most widely used in the inhalers given to asthmatics, and is very effective at preventing asthma attacks if it is taken regularly. It is less effective at relieving symptoms if it is only taken during an attack. It can also be puffed up the nose with the help of a device called an insufflator, and is therefore useful for preventing rhinitis. The drug can also be swallowed in a capsule, and in this form it has proved useful for preventing inflammatory asthma and rashes caused by food allergy, but asthma can often be blocked by inhaling the drug.

6

The Little Children Suffer

You have probably gathered from the preceding chapters that food allergy is a highly controversial subject among doctors. There are some who are unwilling to believe that it affects more than a tiny minority, while there are others who believe that all of us probably have some kind of food allergy. These beliefs influence their diagnoses. A doctor who does not believe that they are common is obviously only going to diagnose food allergy if he is absolutely unable to suggest any other cause. On the other hand, I have sat in the office of an American clinical ecologist and seen him diagnose five consecutive patients who were visiting him for the first time as 'classic cases of food allergy'. When the experts disagree, what are we humble patients to believe?

Ailing Infants

In the coming chapters we shall be looking at the significance of food and chemical allergies in many diseases. As parents of young children are probably those of us most likely to be perplexed and worried by contradictory medical opinions, childhood illness is perhaps the best place to start. Controversy about food allergy is as sharp in this field as in any other; in recent publications one specialist has claimed that food allergy affects less than one child in three hundred, while another declared that it affected more than one child in three!

If we forget these statistics, which are not of much practical use anyway, what do we know about infant food allergy? The main symptoms which affect babies are diarrhoea and vomiting, rashes, asthma, a vulnerability to infections and an apparent inability to thrive and grow. The factors which seem to increase the likelihood of food allergy in infants are having an allergic parent, being bottle-fed with cow's milk, and being introduced to solid foods early in life.

All allergic complaints tend to run in families, though there is no clear pattern of inheritance or any well-understood genetic reason for this. The Canadian paediatrician Dr John Gerrard found that many mothers of children with milk allergies had had similar trouble themselves when they were small, and that one in six still reacted badly to cow's milk. In some types of allergy the cause may be a missing enzyme or enzymes. This explains why Mediterraneans, Asians and black people are generally less able to digest milk: these races have lower amounts of lactase, the enzyme which breaks down milk sugar, than people of European origin.

Breast feeding seems to be the best way of preventing allergic reactions. When a baby is born its immune system is only partly developed. Until now it has been relying on its mother to protect it against infections with her antibodies. Breast milk contains large amounts of the IgA antibody which serves as a first line of defence against foreign proteins. Although cow's milk also contains antibodies, they are of course the kind of antibodies a calf would need. A calf has to be prepared for life as a grass-eating cud-chewer with a very different digestive system from a human child, who faces life as an omnivore.

Human milk and cow's milk do have some proteins in common, though cow's milk contains much more protein than human milk and relatively large amounts of a particular protein, beta-lactoglobulin, which is not present in human milk. It is this protein which babies find especially hard to break down and which therefore presents the greatest risk.

In a provocative article in the *Lancet* of 7 October, 1978, two doctors specializing in tropical medicine, Alan Jackson and Michael Golden, pointed out that cow's milk was designed to encourage a flourishing growth of bacteria in the upper end of the small bowel, the first length of intestine on the way out from the stomach. Human milk, on the other hand, was designed to *discourage* bacteria. Jackson and Golden found that children in Jamaica who had just been weaned onto cow's milk were regularly being brought into their clinic with persistent diarrhoea. Although the symptoms suggested that they had either developed an allergy to the foreign proteins in cow's milk or were unable to break down lactose, the babies responded beautifully to metronidazole, a drug which kills parasitic micro-organisms which flourish in the gut. After a course of treatment with this drug children who had been sickly, undernourished and stunted began to thrive on cow's milk without suffering any of their former symptoms.

In other words, there are three main reasons why a child might not be able to tolerate cow's milk. Firstly, it contains proteins which cannot be broken down and which may therefore stimulate cells to produce the IgE antibodies which cause inflammation. Secondly, the child may lack the lactase enzyme which breaks down lactose. And thirdly, as Jackson and Golden found, cow's milk may encourage the growth of harmful micro-organisms.

Of course we are still left with this question: Why don't all babies react badly to cow's milk? Some pundits would say that they do react badly, but some react more noticeably than others. This idea is highly controversial. Most babies who are bottle-fed seem to grow into healthy children, even though as babies they are more likely than breast-fed babies to fall victim to infections and allergies.

The gravest accusation which has been levelled at cow's milk is that it is responsible for 'cot death', the sudden death which strikes some babies for no apparent reason. In 1960 a report in the *Lancet* claimed that cot death could be caused by an anaphylactic reaction to cow's milk.

Bad news about cow's milk is bound to distress those mothers who cannot breast-feed their children. Breast feeding is sometimes impossible if the mother is ill, if she has an insufficient supply of milk in her breasts, if her nipples become cracked or sore, or if she has to take medicines which could be passed to her baby through her milk. Moreover, if a baby does not have enough lactase it may find its mother's milk indigestible, because human milk contains even more lactose than cow's milk.

Artificial milks are available to feed children who cannot be breast-fed, and there are enzyme preparations, such as the American product Lact-aid, which can be added to cow's milk to break down the lactose into glucose and galactose, which can be assimilated easily. Artificial milks are based on meat or vegetable products and provide the proteins a child would get from milk.

Although some races are more prone to lactose intolerance, it is a problem which affects adults more than newborn babies. It can be inherited, but it can also result from infections and disorders which damage the stomach linings.

The symptoms of lactose intolerance are very similar to those of other problems caused by milk, but it is not very hard to distinguish between them. The patient goes on a lactose-free diet until the symptoms have disappeared, and is then challenged with lactose to see if they return. If the symptoms do not disappear, it is reasonable to assume that lactose is not causing them or is only partly to blame.

Artificial milks are only necessary for long-term infant feeding if the baby cannot take human or cow's milk. And they too have their problems. One of the most popular artificial milks is made from soya beans. It was first introduced in 1929, at a time when soya beans did not form a very significant part of the Western diet and were not thought to be allergenic. Over the past ten years, however, allergy to soya beans has been seen more and more in children and adults. It is still less common than milk allergy, but we might wonder whether the increase in soya bean allergy has anything to do with the growing presence of soya bean products in popular processed foods.

If a mother cannot give breast milk, there are other sources for this valuable product. Some hospitals have 'milk banks' which hold milk donated by mothers who produce more than their own babies need. In the past it was common for wealthier women to hand their children over to wet nurses. These were usually women who had had children of their own and whose breasts had been kept in practice by constant use over the years. Fashion seems to be against wet nurses these days, which is a pity, because a generous bosom surely offers more than any plastic nipple. But of course fashion does not obey laws of common sense.

In the *Lancet* article which I mentioned earlier, Dr Jackson and Dr Golden concluded that 'The use of formulas based on cow's milk should be restricted — particularly in infants under six months, who depend heavily on passive immunity and in whom active immunity is at a critical stage of development — to situations where there is no alternative.' They went on to say that 'The properties and use of alternative milks to those of ruminants should be explored.'

Although they make no specific suggestions as to where these milks might be obtained, this idea has possibilities which take us far beyond anything conceived by dietitians past or present. Baboon milk is one alternative which springs immediately to mind. The baboon is much more similar to the human than the cow, and perhaps we would find that its milk was more nutritious and less allergenic. And if ancient legend is to be believed, Romulus and Remus, the founders of Roman civilization, were suckled by a she-wolf!

Seriously, such exotic sources of food look rather more plausible when we consider how much our infant feeding habits have changed during the past fifty years. According to Dr S. J. Fomon's authoritative textbook *Infant Nutrition*, European and American mothers until the 1920s never used to feed their children solid foods before they were at least a year old. The fashion is completely different today, when children are weaned onto solids at a few months. Feeding habits have undergone a revolution unmatched by an evolutionary change in ourselves.

The British clinical ecologist Dr Richard Mackarness has put forward a theory that evolution of the human species has not moved fast enough to keep up with our ever changing diet. He believes that fresh meat and vegetables are the least allergenic foods because they are the ones which formed the natural diet of Stone Age folk living in the wild. We now live on a diet of refined grains and sugars which our metabolism is not designed to handle. He has found that patients with psychiatric illness get better when refined cereals are taken out of their diet, and his 'Stone Age diet', consisting of meat, animal fat and fresh vegetables ad lib, but without refined sugar and grains, has helped many obese people lose weight.

Nevertheless, although his evolutionary theory may hold true for some adults, it does not really fit with the kind of food allergies suffered by young chilen. Cereals, certainly, are one of the most common causes of food allergy in chilen, but if we survey the scientific literature about food allergy, we find that eggs, fish, tomatoes, oranges, bananas and nuts are blamed just as often. These foods would feature large in a natural prehistoric diet and we could hardly blame evolution for an allergy to any of them.

Allergy to these foods is often harder to detect than milk allergy because by the time a child is eating such things its diet will be mixed. Cow's milk allergy is easy to detect because milk is probably the only thing a very young child is consuming. However, specialists appear to agree that allergies to solid foods are much commoner among babies under one year old than among older children. In some, the allergy may persist into later life; in others it will pass. Quite often, though, an allergy to a food may disappear, only to be replaced a year or two later by an allergy to pollen or some other substance.

Bed-wetting

'If this problem is caused by allergy, it is most uncommon.' Doris Rapp, MD, and A. W. Frankland, MD, *Allergies: Questions and Answers.*

The comment above would be the typical orthodox medical answer to anyone who asked whether food allergy or any kind of allergy made children wet the bed. The fact that it comes from two eminent allergists who have devoted much attention to food allergy might make one think that the idea merited little more discussion.

Bed-wetting (the medical name is enuresis) is only regarded as a medical problem if a child persistently wets the bed after the age of three, by which time most children have learned to control their bladder. Though inflammation of the bladder is sometimes acknowledged to be the cause, it is usually attributed to emotional problems, which the child will eventually overcome. Doctors generally advise parents not to scold children who wet the bed, because this often makes them do it all the more. Sometimes electrical gadgets are used to train the child out of the habit; they consist of an alarm bell or buzzer wired to a simple circuit which is switched on by the first drop of urine to leak from the unfortuate youngster. The alarm wakes the child and thereby alerts it to the imminent flood.

Despite almost universal acceptance of the 'emotional'

explanation for bed-wetting, a handful of specialists resolutely maintain that food allergy is not only *a* cause but *the* principal cause of the problem. And they have produced persuasive evidence to back their argument.

Bed-wetting is not just an affliction of childhood. Adults suffer too, not just old people who are beginning to lose control over their bladders, but ordinary young and middle-aged grown-ups. As long ago as 1923 the American allergist W. W. Duke identified flour and certain vegetables as the cause of painful bladder complaints, and in the 1930s the British allergist George Bray used elimination diets to diagnose food allergies as the cause of adult bed-wetting. They were only able to find a few cases, however, and their report fell on deaf ears. It was not until 1957 that Dr J. C. Breneman, now a leading American allergist, documented his investigation of sixty-five bed-wetters, all of whom had overcome their problem as soon as certain foods were eliminated from their diets. Breneman did not stop at this; he did biopsies of these patients' bladders and found that their bladder lining was invariably swollen like the nasal mucosa of someone suffering from allergic rhinitis. Their urine contained large quantities of eosinophils, a type of white cell whose function is still unexplained but which is strongly associated with allergic disease. Since then Dr Breneman has cured several hundred bed-wetters with the help of elimination diets, and now claims that food allergy is responsible for the complaint in four cases out of five. He also claims that treatment of their food allergy also immediately relieved the various psychiatric ills to which some of these patients were victim.

In his book *Basics of Food Allergy* he offers an amusing diagnostic aid for food allergy and bed-wetting. Men and boys who are allergic to milk and who also wet the bed display a positive Chvostek reflex. In other words, when you tap the skin over the facial nerve on their cheek, the muscles in the upper lip and cheek contract sharply into a one-sided grimace. This reaction recurs consistently in males who are allergic to milk. 'If the reflex is found in adults,' he suggests, 'ask the simple question "at what age did you stop wetting the bed?" Frequently there will be utter amazement and the reply: "How did you know?" '

The Chvostek reflex has been attributed to calcium deficiency, though this idea has been disputed. Whatever its origin, Dr Breneman finds that the reflex will persist sometimes for years after the bed-wetting has stopped.

The other leading proponent of the food allergy/bed-wetting syndrome is the Canadian paediatrician John Gerrard, a professor at the University of Saskatchewan. The first clue he found to link the two phenomena came from his supervising a number of children who were suffering from asthma and gastrointestinal problems caused by cow's milk allergy. One of his boy patients had a sister who wet the bed. The boy responded well to a milk-free diet and for the sake of domestic convenience his mother had given the sister the same food. Once off milk and dairy products she stopped her bed-wetting. The little girl was quite happy to give up her milk, but was still tempted by ice-cream. Unfortunately, shortly after eating some she wet herself — and got a thrashing from her father.

Professor Gerrard and his colleagues have since discovered that bed-wetting children have a small bladder capacity. Their bladder is small because of a muscle spasm which disappears when certain foods are taken out of their diet.

Foods are not the only cause. He has also come across children who wet themselves after being exposed to house dust, cigarette smoke or pollen. One child shared an allergy to maple pollen with her father: she would begin to wet herself on the same day as her father got hay fever.

Heredity plays an even more noticeable role in enuresis than in other allergic complaints. From his studies of many families Gerrard has found that almost half the parents of enuretic children had themselves been bed-wetters. There was a one-in-four chance that siblings of enuretic children would be enuretic too.

The complaint can be relieved by antihistamines or by imipramine, one of the tricyclic drugs more commonly used to treat depression. Their effects are seldom more than temporary, however, and diet appears to be the most reliable way of getting rid of the disease for good. If enuresis is being caused by an allergen, it is worth taking trouble to isolate it, because the Saskatchewan doctors have found that enuretic girls are more vulnerable to recurrent urinary infections like cystitis later in life.

7

Coeliac Disease — Inherited or Ingested?

Milk allergy in infancy can lead to a disorder which is much more worrying than cystitis. One child in ten will go on to develop coeliac disease, a chronic complaint in which damage to the lining of the intestine prevents the body from absorbing fats, calcium and other important nutrients. Coeliac (which literally means 'belly') disease was once thought to be a transient childhood disease, but it is now recognized to be a permanent condition which persists through adult life. Recent estimates suggest that about one person in seven hundred suffers from coeliac disease, though the figure has been rising steadily since the 1950s, when doctors really began to interest themselves in the condition and actively look out for it.

The symptoms of coeliac disease are loss of weight, diarrhoea with pulpy, smelly stools which are full of undigested fat, a stomach which puffs up and causes pain, and sometimes vomiting. The symptoms are caused by an intolerance to gluten, a protein found in wheat, rye, barley and oats. There are three main theories for this intolerance: it could be (1) an abnormal immunological reaction to the protein; (2) a deficiency of peptidase enzyme, which results in partially broken down toxic material damaging the intestine; or (3) an abnormality in the membranes in the gut which allows the protein to stick to the intestine lining. It could even be a combination of such mechanisms. For instance, partially broken-down protein particles could stick in the gut lining, where their presence would attract the attention of antibody-producing white cells, which would in turn lead to inflammation and damage to the intestine.

Dr Samuel Gee of St Bartholomew's Hospital, London, was the first physician to realize that what he called 'the coeliac affection' was causing malnutrition and sometimes death in young children.

He described the symptoms of the disease in 1888, and thought that it might be curable by excluding wheat and other cereal products from the diet. 'If the patient be cured at all, it must be by means of diet. The allowance of farinaceous food must be small', he wrote.

In 1950 a Dutch doctor, W. K. Dicke, identified gluten as the ingredient which was to blame, and his research led to the use of gluten-free diets by people with coeliac disease. Since then another ingredient of cereals, alpha-gliadin, and a number of substances created by the breakdown of cereals in the stomach have also been shown to be potentially harmful, but gluten still seems to be the ringleader.

Coeliac disease is now classified as a permanent condition which can be relieved but not cured by withdrawal of gluten. The most important diagnostic test is a biopsy of the small intestine. It can be a gruelling experience for the patient, who has to swallow a capsule about an inch long and attached to a polythene tube. With the help of an X-ray monitor, the doctor watches the capsule and tube descend down the oesophagus into the stomach. The patient has to keep gulping away until the capsule is coaxed through into the small intestine. The end of the capsule is then allowed to sink into the mucous membrane lining the intestine. The doctor then pulls on a wire in the polythene tube, which activates a cutting device in the capsule. The capsule, together with the sample of mucous membrane it has snipped off, is then pulled out. In a healthy person the intestinal lining is covered with little structures which under a microscope look like fronds or fingers or the tentacles of a sea anemone, and which are called *villi*. If you are suffering from coeliac disease these villi will have disappeared. If you go on a gluten-free diet, the villi will grow back; they will disappear again if you relapse from the diet.

As with almost any condition, some people suffer more acutely than others from coeliac disease. An infant who is constantly sick, bloated, the victim of diarrhoea and who does not grow, quickly attracts attention. But many older children and adult coeliacs are only diagnosed after they have come to their doctor with anaemia, rickets or some other complaint which is due to their inability to absorb essential nutrients through their damaged gut.

The origin of the disease is still a puzzle. One in ten coeliacs has a very close relative who also suffers. And you may remember from Chapter 3 that coeliacs have a very much higher than average chance of having a parent, sibling or child who suffers from migraine, asthma, eczema, epilepsy, schizophrenia or other mental illness. So there seems to be a strong hereditary factor involved in coeliac disease and other diseases associated with food allergy.

But to what extent can the disease actually be brought on by a food? Dr Anne Ferguson, an Edinburgh physician and authority on coeliac disease, claims that the development of coeliac disease may be made more likely if gluten is given early in life or if the patient has had milk allergy. She has noticed that young coeliacs lack the protective IgA antibody and are thus less able to deal with allergic proteins.

Can all these things be blamed on inherited defects, or are they really the result of feeding a child with foreign proteins which it is not ready to accept? There is some evidence that coeliac disease may be caused by diet. Some infants have all the symptoms of coeliac disease — bloating, diarrhoea, poor growth and destroyed villi — and get completely better after going on a gluten-free diet. But if a year or two later they start eating gluten foods again, they do not relapse as a coeliac would. They remain healthy. This so-called 'transient gluten intolerance' has only been seen in very young children. It is quite conceivable that if they had not been diagnosed in the nick of time their condition would have progressed until it was irreversible. The development of the disease could depend on an inherited vulnerability aggravated by regular exposure to gluten.

A gluten-free diet is one of the hardest to follow, and anyone who needs detailed advice would do well to consult the Coeliac Society, a patients' association based in London (PO Box 181, London NW2 2QY. Telephone 01-459-2440).

The reason many people on gluten-free diets do not get completely better is that they are still inadvertently consuming gluten. In a report in the *British Medical Journal* in 1975, Dr P. G. Baker claimed that 65 per cent of patients on gluten-free diets were in fact eating 'hidden' gluten. International standards set by the World Health Organization do not lay down any upper limit to the gluten content of supposedly gluten-free products. They only say that these products may contain wheat, rye, barley or oat flour from which all gluten has, *so far as practicable,* been extracted.

A coeliac patient only has to ingest a very small amount of gluten to jeopardize his or her health. Indeed, some go as far as providing their priest with gluten-free communion wafers. Indigestion tablets, one might think, would not be likely to present a risk; but the manufacturers of the antacid Nulacin, which contains gluten, feel obliged to warn coeliac patients against using their product.

We have seen how official committees responsible for medicines are prepared to let tartrazine, a proven allergen, be added to drugs intended for asthmatics, so it is perhaps hardly surprising that an even more cavalier attitude prevails towards foods.

8

Hyperactive Children

Is your child overactive, disruptive, compulsive, irritable, reckless, excitable, impulsive, easily frustrated, demanding? Does he or she have poor concentration, or do much worse at school than a child with his or her intelligence should?

Most parents would have to admit that their little darlings were just occasionally all these things. You would probably be worried if they *didn't* go a little wild now and then. But if they are like this all the time, pausing only now and then for a bout of acute misery and lethargy, then something must have gone wrong.

A severely hyperactive child is a constant trial to parents, teachers and anyone else who has to look after it. Hyperactivity appears to be on the increase, especially in the cities of the United States, and psychologists are bewildered by it. A common medical treatment is a prescription of the stimulant drug Ritalin. On the face of it, you might think that a stimulant was the last thing to give a hyperactive child, but apparently it works by making the child pay more attention to detail, by replacing excitability with obsessiveness. The disadvantage is that it dulls imagination as well as physical exuberance.

Drug treatment is a poor substitute for eliminating the cause of the problem. But what is the cause of hyperactivity? Some psychiatrists blame it on an unstable family background. Unfortunately, even if this is the case, such domestic problems are often impossible to cure. Some pundits have even blamed hyperactivity on television, though no one has shown that hyperactivity can be cured by switching the set off for a few weeks. Of course, both these approaches are based on the assumption that the problem is caused by something fed into the child's mind.

Perhaps it would be more profitable to look at things fed into the child's body instead.

I have already briefly described how clinical ecologists have proved that many mental complaints can be caused by allergy to foods, spores and chemicals. In his 1975 publication *Can Your Child Read?* the American paediatrician William Crook documented case histories of children whose academic performance increased markedly after allergenic foods had been taken out of their diet. Dr Ben Feingold has blamed food dyes for causing hyperactivity and found that a number of chemicals in the atmosphere or added to foods affect the way in which the body absorbs essential trace elements. Dr E. Lodge-Rees, a San Francisco physician who specializes in treating psychiatrically disturbed children and adolescents, has found high levels of aluminium — which usually originates from cooking pots and cooking foil — in the blood and tissues of delinquent children as well as in adult psychiatric patients. Professor Derek Bryce-Smith of Reading University has drawn a correlation between atmospheric lead pollution in Glasgow and the unusually high incidence of mental retardation among children in the most polluted areas of that city. Lead in the tissues reduces the body's ability to absorb zinc, an essential trace element which the body uses to activate about forty different enzymes. Animal experiments have shown that the offspring of mothers with abnormally low zinc levels were mentally sluggish, found it hard to learn and had little resistance to stress.

Lead poisoning was a quite common occupational hazard in the nineteenth century, when the metal was used widely in industry with little thought for the need to protect workers from exposure to it. The problem with lead is that the body has no way of getting rid of it; it accumulates, especially in the bones. The symptoms are variable: many people suffer from sharp abdominal pains; others may become anaemic or suffer brain and nerve damage. Treatment consists of giving large doses of calcium to strengthen the bones; calcium may also succeed in dislodging accumulated lead. There are also synthetic substances called chelating agents available which surround the molecules of metal and are then excreted, taking the metal with them.

Industrial pollution does account for some of the lead in the atmosphere today, but the principal source is petrol engine exhaust fumes. In 1971 the journal *Science* reported how tigers in the Staten Island Zoo in New York had died or fallen ill because of the high levels of lead in the urban air they were breathing. In Britain high levels of lead have been found in people living near the 'Spaghetti Junction' motorway intersection in Birmingham and other places where there is a lot of traffic.

Lead used in household paints presents a threat to many young children who have pica, an inexplicable craving for unnatural food. Pica means 'magpie', and its commonest manifestation is in infants who develop a taste for pieces of coal or earth. They may also pick off flakes of peeling paint and eat them. Laws now restrict the use of lead in paints, though plenty of old, dilapidated houses present babies with a treasure trove of tasty paint morsels. In 1970 the New York health authorities had become so concerned about this kind of poisoning that they embarked on a screening programme. In that year alone they identified 2,600 cases of lead poisoning in infants. If it is not caught early, lead poisoning gives young children irreversible brain damage.

Another possible cause of lead poisoning in adults is moonshine liquor, especially popular in the South in the United States and in Irish communities in Britain. This hazard was recognized more than 250 years ago when the elders of the Massachusetts Bay Colony banned the use of pewter stills for distilling rum, because lead contamination in the booze was giving drinkers 'the dry gripes'. Moonshiners no longer use pewter, but they do use lead-based solders for joining their still pipes and, according to a report in *Scientific American* in 1971, use old automobile radiators containing lead as condensers!

The toxic effect of lead and other heavy metals such as mercury, cadmium and arsenic are well known. Much less recognized are the potential hazards of 'permitted' chemicals which go into food and drink.

The yellow dye tartrazine was the first common additive to be blamed for allergic reactions such as asthma and rashes. Since then, almost every synthetic dye and flavouring agent used in processed food and drink has been identified as an occasional cause of such problems, even though their chemical structures are different.

People who are sensitive to dyes and flavourings, especially tartrazine, tend to be sensitive to aspirin too. Aspirin manufactured today is a synthetic product, but it is chemically related to the salicylate chemicals which occur naturally in almonds, apples, oranges and several other fruits. Some people who are allergic to aspirin have to give up these fruits to remain well.

Hyperactivity, we might think, has little in common with asthma and rashes. Nevertheless, it does now seem that some hyperactive children can be cured by a diet which eliminates all salicylates and artifical dyes and colourings. The leading light in this kind of treatment has been Dr Ben Feingold, chief allergist at the Kaiser Permanente Medical Center in San Francisco, California. He does not claim that foods and additives are the only cause of hyperactivity, but he offers some interesting case histories which all but prove that they play an important part.

A seven-year-old boy who was referred to his clinic had been severely hyperactive for several years. At home he 'stomped around, slamming the doors and kicking the walls and even charging oncoming cars with his bicycle'. At school his hyperactive behaviour was disruptive, resulting in his inability to learn.

The boy had been taken to see numerous paediatricians as well as neurologists, psychiatrists and psychologists, and had even undergone an exhaustive medical and neurological survey. 'Nothing succeeded,' Dr Feingold reports, 'until the child was placed on a salicylate-free diet, which eliminated natural salicylate-containing foods and all foods and drinks with artificial colours and flavours. After a few weeks of dietary control, the child became well adjusted at home and at school. Whenever he broke the rules of the diet, his hyperactive behaviour would return almost immediately.'

Another seven-year-old with similar problems had already been taking Ritalin for eighteen months before he was referred to the allergy clinic and put on the same diet. Two weeks later his schoolteachers told his mother that his reading ability had markedly improved. When Dr Feingold learned this, he halved the boy's daily dose of Ritalin and encouraged him to keep up the diet. Three weeks later his mother reported that his behaviour at home and school had improved almost beyond measure, and he was taken off the drug altogether. Within the next three weeks his teachers were saying that he was the best reader in his class, that his writing had also improved remarkably and that he was going to be promoted to a higher grade.

Salicylates and food additives are not the only dietary factors. Milk, Dr Feingold says, heads the list of common foods which are associated with hyperactivity. This has been borne out by clinical trials conducted by two Massachusetts doctors, James O'Shea and Seymour Porter.

The purpose of their study was to determine, using double-blind methods, whether children's hyperactive behaviour could be switched on and switched off by giving them skin injections or sublingual doses of foods, food additives and airborne allergens such as pollen and moulds. They selected fifteen children, aged between five and thirteen, who were believed by their parents and teachers to be in need of treatment for hyperactivity and poor learning ability.

In the tests the children were given injections into the skin of tiny amounts of foods and airborne allergens (0.05 millilitres of an extract containing one part in 100). The dyes were given under the tongue, and in very dilute form. The children were then observed by a psychologist for any significant change in their behaviour.

Dyes provoked reactions in almost all of them: thirteen out of fifteen reacted to the red dye, and twelve to the yellow and blue dyes; eleven reacted to milk; seven to peanuts and/or tomato; six to apple, cane sugar, corn or orange; five to chocolate; four to wheat; and three to egg. Dust, mould and pollen extracts only caused reactions in a few.

When the tests showed that the child was apparently sensitive to a food or dye, switch-off injections or drops or a placebo of water were given. The children then went back to their homes and schools, where they were carefully watched by their parents and teachers, who did not know whether they had been given the 'switch-off' or a placebo.

The switch-offs generally worked well. Reports from three quarters of the parents and more than half the teachers showed that the switch-off had had a significantly more beneficial effect than the placebo. In other words, there was reasonable evidence not only that foods and chemicals could cause hyperactive behaviour, but also that this behaviour could be prevented. Switch-off drops and injections may not be as reliable as diets, but if they do work, they should be very useful for children who are not easily kept to diets.

Dr Feingold has observed five common features associated with the condition of hyperactivity:

1. This kind of disturbed behaviour occurs almost exclusively in boys.
2. Usually only one child in a family is involved.
3. Most but not all of the children have a family history of allergy.
4. The children are usually of normal or high IQ.
5. Their regular diet contains large quantities of food additives.

These facts may not bring us any nearer to understanding the cause of the affliction, but some of them coincide with the features of other allergic diseases. Asthma, for instance, affects more boys than girls. And we know that a family history of allergy increases the chances that a child will have some kind of allergic disease. All this brings us back to the question raised by coeliac disease: To what extent is the disease inherited and to what extent is it created?

Dr Feingold has pointed out that the increase in hyperactivity in children corresponds historically with the increase in the use of food additives. This observation does not prove anything; if it did we could equally well say that heart disease was caused by television since the increase in heart disease corresponds well with the increase in TV sales! Nevertheless it is circumstantial evidence which strengthens the case.

If diet is involved in hyperactivity, it is not necessarily the child's diet which is to blame. We know that many drugs taken by a pregnant mother can pass into the unborn child and into breast milk. The same must be true of the chemical additives in foods. If so, the mother's diet may lay the foundations of trouble to come.

9
Migraine and Mental Disorders

All that comes from milk increases melancholy.
— Robert Burton, *The Anatomy of Melancholy*, 1651

Philosophers did us a great disservice when they suggested that mind and body were separate phenomena. Leaving aside its religious and moral implications, this bizarre concept has been largely responsible for the notion that mental disease was somehow different from physical disease. It is only very recently that mental disease began to lose its stigma and become regarded as something which you did not have to be ashamed of.

Emotional distress has a direct effect on our physical functions, and physical distress can upset our minds. When a patient has been suffering for a long time, it can be difficult to distinguish between cause and effect. People suffering from pain usually become depressed if the condition persists. Depression also lowers their intolerance to pain, so they may be acutely distressed by a complaint which a happier person would shrug off.

I have already described cases which show that there is a definite link between food and chemical allergy and a whole spectrum of mental disorders. All too often foods are the last thing a doctor suspects, and patients are unfairly branded as 'neurotic' when they fail to respond to conventional treatment. This is well illustrated by the case of a traffic warden who suffered terribly from migraine and depression. Her doctor, Ronald Finn, suggested that she should give up chocolate and cheese. She did so, and her migraines disappeared. Her depression did not go, however, and her bouts of melancholy became so frequent and intense that her superiors were considering whether she should be dismissed from her job as mentally unfit. Dr Finn then suggested that she should try giving up wheat foods. Three weeks later she was completely better, and on a wheat-free diet her misery has not returned.

Migraine is not classified as a mental disorder, but it is widely believed that stress, tension and worry are often responsible for bringing on migraine attacks in many sufferers. We have already seen how food and chemicals can induce mental distress, and it is now beginning to look as though food allergy may be the cause of the psychological upsets which are sometimes associated with migraine.

A few years ago the British migraine specialist Dr Edda Hannington discovered that a proportion of migraine patients would have attacks after eating foods which contained a particular amino acid called tyramine. Tyramine is found in chocolate, cheese, broad beans, yeast and meat extracts and red wine, and migraineurs learn to avoid these foods. It seems that they lack the enzyme monoamine oxidase, which breaks down tyramine and prevents excessive quantities of it accumulating in the blood. However, experiments designed to keep up sufferers' tyramine levels did not succeed in getting rid of their migraines. So researchers started looking for other explanations.

Although few specialists disagree with the idea that certain foods can bring on migraine, they point out that foods which do not contain tyramine can also induce migraine attacks. Dr Ellen Grant of London's Charing Cross Hospital has claimed that the contraceptive pill is causing food allergies in women and that these allergies are manifesting themselves as migraine. She has found that a significant number of women patients lose their migraine if they give up the Pill. When she subsequently put these women on an exclusion diet which made them avoid foods to which they had evidence of allergy, their migraines disappeared altogether.

Food allergies tend to develop after a woman has been on the Pill for about two years, Dr Grant observes. Cigarette smokers are also likely to develop food allergies, but with them the allergies only become noticeable after they have been smoking for twenty years or so. Dr Grant's opinion is based on her experience of several hundred patients who were referred to her migraine and headache clinics during the past years. She noticed that a surprisingly high proportion of these patients were either women taking oral contraceptives, or men who had been smoking for most of their lives. She also found that ergotamine, a drug used to treat migraine, appeared to be doing more harm than good to many of her patients. Although the drug worked well at first, prolonged use resulted in migraine actually getting worse. This observation has been confirmed by other British migraine specialists, who now advise their colleagues not to prescribe ergotamine.

If her patients were able to give up the Pill, smoking or ergotamine, many would lose their headaches. Most of her patients, however, were either unwilling or unable to give them up, so she suggested that they should try avoiding cheese, chocolate, citrus fruits, alcohol, excessive stress and even hunger, which might trigger attacks by upsetting their body chemistry. Non-smokers were also advised to avoid inhaling other people's cigarette smoke. This advice proved beneficial. By following it more than half the smokers, a third of the women on the Pill and a small proportion of the ergotamine patients and patients who did not take any of these drugs lost their headaches.

These results were gratifying, but Dr Grant wondered whether more patients could be helped by excluding other foods from their diet. She therefore persuaded all of them to go on a strict simple diet for five days to clear possible allergens from their system, and then to feed themselves common foods one at a time to see if they got any adverse reaction to them. The simple diet she recommended consisted of lamb and pears, washed down with bottled spring water. She had been suggested this diet by the British clinical ecologist Dr John Mansfield, who had found that lamb and pears were among the foods least likely to be the cause of allergy.

Forty foods were included in the feeding tests, and patients were not allowed to take more than three new foods on any one day, and had to leave a space of several hours before trying each item. Their reaction to each food was assessed by a pulse test and by recording all other unpleasant symptoms which followed eating. A few patients did actually get headaches after eating some foods, but the commonest adverse reactions were a racing pulse, 'bloating', or other stomach upsets. Very nearly all the patients reacted badly to several foods; some reacted to only one or two, others reacted to as many as thirty, though the average was about ten.

Everyone was advised to give up eating all the foods which had produced a reaction. The foods which had most frequently been identified were wheat products (in 78 per cent of patients); oranges (65 per cent); eggs (45 per cent); tea and coffee (each 40 per cent); chocolate and milk (each 37 per cent): beef (35 per cent); corn, cane sugar and yeast (each 33 per cent); mushrooms (30 per cent); and peas (28 per cent). Patients who followed the exclusion diet did amazingly well: 85 per cent of them suffered no more headaches or migraine, and all the others experienced a great reduction in their suffering.

Although exclusion diets seem to have worked better than any other therapy, Dr Grant believes that it is better to prevent food allergies developing in the first place, and she now speaks out vigorously against oral contraceptives and smoking. She does not know exactly how food allergies are caused by these things, but like other clinical ecologists she suggests that they may be having a variety of effects on hormones, enzymes and other subtle aspects of body chemistry which gradually upset its natural balance and produce intolerances.

Migrainous neuralgia is a particularly unpleasant kind of headache which causes its sufferers even worse pain than more common forms of migraine. It tends to strike its victims spasmodically: they may go for months without an attack, but then be stricken with bouts of paroxysmal headaches which occur several times a day and last for up to two hours at a time. The pain is usually on one side of the front of the head and may also affect the eye and cause weeping and a runny nose. According to the medical textbooks the causes of migrainous neuralgia are unknown, but one of Dr Finn's cases suggests that food may be a culprit here too. His patient, an otherwise healthy middle-aged man, suffered so badly from his attacks that he would yell and moan out loud and bang his head against the wall. Wondering whether cheese and chocolate, two of the patient's favourite foods, were involved, Dr Finn suggested that he should give them up as an experiment. He did and has not suffered since.

By far the most impressive evidence linking migraine with food came from researchers at the Hospital for Sick Children in Great

Ormond Street in 1983. They studied over 80 children for several months, beginning by giving them a very simple diet to which they gradually added extra items one by one. Foods were specially prepared (with the help of food companies Heinz and Kelloggs) so that the young patients would not know whether they actually contained a particular ingredient or not.

Reporting their findings in the *Lancet* the doctors revealed that an enormous variety of different foods could cause migraine in different children. The table below lists the foods the doctors tested for and the percentage of children for whom these foods caused problems. As you see, eggs, cheese and chocolate came top of the list.

Table VI

CHILDREN IN WHOM FOODS CAUSED SYMPTOMS

	%		%		%		%
Cow's milk	67	Soya	17	Chicken	under 8	Veg oils	under 5
Egg	60	Tea	17	White wht flr	"	Lentils	"
Chocolate	55	Oats	15	Artifical milk	"	Peas	"
Orange	52	Goat's milk	15	Banana	"	Ice cream	"
Wheat	52	Coffee	15	Strawberries	"	Rabbit	1 person only
Benzoic acid	35	Peanuts	12	Melon	"	Date	"
Cheese	32	Bacon		Carrots	"	Avocado	"
Tomato	32	Potato	10	Lamb	under 5	Rhubarb	"
Tartrazine	30	Yeast	10	Rice	"	Leek	"
Rye	30	Mixed nuts	10	Malt	"	Lettuce	"
Fish	22	Apple	10	Sugar	"	Cucumber	"
Pork	22	Peaches	10	Ginger	"	Cauliflower	"
Beef	22	Grapes	10	Honey	"	Mushrooms	"
Maize	22			Pineapple	"	Runner beans	"

They found that some children might get an attack quite soon after eating a particular food, while others would not get an attack for several hours. Children were usually very fond of the foods which gave them migraine. However the doctors did find that even when a child reacted badly to a large number of foods it was possible to devise a diet which avoided those foods. In fact one child reacted to twenty-four different foods, but they still managed to work out a diet which left out all those foods and banished his migraines altogether.

In the April 1978 issue of the *Lancet*, Professor J. W. T. Dickerson and his colleagues at the University of Surrey provided another example of a food allergy masquerading as a 'stress disease'.

The patient, a man aged 40, had a seven-year history of intermittent abdominal distension and catarrh. The catarrh, often accompanied by a frontal headache, occurred every ten days or so. The symptoms had been thought due to business stress. Common environmental allergens had been excluded. He was put on an exclusion diet and remained symptom-free until bread was included. He had some response on the day after its inclusion, but on the second day the response — catarrh, headache and abdominal distension — was so severe that he had to cease work. Subsequent tests showed that this patient also reacted badly to rye products (Ryvita) and to some extent to bacon. He has now been in good health for nine months, on a diet in which foods made from gluten-free and barley flour have been substituted for wheat products.

Throughout this book we have seen that allergic reactions to foods often resemble complaints which are more usually attributed to stress or anxiety. Stomach upsets, ulcers, palpitations, headaches, inexplicable aches and pains — all these afflictions can be brought on by worry, and I am certainly not suggestinging that food allergy always plays a part in them. Indeed, it is quite possible for stress to provoke intolerance to food. In his textbook *Basics of Food Allergy* Dr Breneman suggests that mental or physical stress may aggravate food intolerance. He writes, 'Patients who are unable to eat fish, for example, in their everyday life situation may find that they can tolerate fish very well during a happy vacation. A less severely fish-allergic patient may tolerate fish in day-to-day life, but then cannot eat fish during a menstrual period or during an episode of marital disharmony.' He and other allergists point out that infections, especially viral infections like hepatitis and influenza, often lead to the patient developing a food allergy.

In his book *Not All in the Mind* Dr Richard Mackarness documented in great detail the case of Joanna, a young mother who had been diagnosed as schizophrenic. She suffered from fits of uncontrollable behaviour in which she would scratch and cut herself mercilessly. She would also turn on her family: on one occasion she had knocked her three-year-old son unconscious, and another time she had thrown her young daughter out of a window.

She was found to be allergic to several foods and got better when they were taken out of her diet. If she ate them again she went into rapid mental decline, becoming depressed, apathetic, and sometimes prone to hallucinations.

The term schizophrenia covers a variety of severe disturbances of perception and behaviour. It was once called dementia praecox (literally 'precocious dementia') because it was most commonly seen in young adults. The popular idea of a schizophrenic being a person with a dual personality, like Dr Jekyll, is rather misleading. The schizophrenic's problem is that he or she cannot distinguish reality from fantasy and lives in a dream or nightmare. Schizophrenics experience delusions and hallucinations and lose their sense of identity; they may refer to themselves as 'he' or 'she' rather than 'I', or laugh out loud while describing an intense physical pain or a gruesome event in their life.

The causes of schizophrenia are the subject of sharp controversy. Theorists are now divided into two camps, those who believe that the disease is biological and those who believe that its causes are social. The 'social' theorists claim that schizophrenia is a psychological reaction to an absurd and disturbing society and family life, and that 'insane' people are really no more ill than the people who call them mad because they find their behaviour undesirable. The 'biological' theorists put forward a variety of explanations to suggest how the disease is caused by abnormalities of body chemistry.

The social approach to schizophrenia is like the Freudian psycholanalytic approach to other mental illnesses. The therapist tries to guide the patient and give him insight into his predicament. But, also like psychoanalysis, the treatment may last for years without producing much in the way of a cure.

The biological camp is divided within itself. There are several kinds of chemical abnormality which have been seen in schizophrenics. None of them seems to explain every aspect of the disease, though each may be a partial explanation of this complex condition.

Excessive amounts of certain substances, notably dopamine and endorphins, have been found in schizophrenics. Most of the drugs used to treat schizophrenics work by blocking the 'receptors' in brain cells where dopamine normally attaches itself. Endorphins are part of the body's own system for controlling pain, though this is almost certainly just a small part of their total function. They are not related chemically to morphine and the other opiate drugs, but their effects are similar. Schizophrenics have been found to have unusually high amounts of endorphins in their spinal fluid, and their symptoms have sometimes been relieved by giving them a dose of naloxone, a drug which dislodges morphine and endorphins from their receptors.

Schizophrenia is also associated with a deficiency of prostaglandins and of melatonin, a substance produced by the pineal gland, situated at the front of the brain just above and between the eyes.

Other recent theories say that schizophrenia is the result of insufficient quantities of the trace element zinc, caused by chemical poisoning which prevents the body from absorbing zinc properly, or by a lack of zinc in the diet. The theories which perhaps come closest to the main theme of this book are that schizophrenia is caused by an allergy to wheat or by an abnormal immunological reaction to several food antigens.

All these ideas are based on research findings rather than mere speculation, and they are complementary rather than contradictory. In other words, they are not false, but neither are they complete explanations. They are different aspects of the same thing. Although I shall concentrate on the food factors of the disease, we shall see that these do in fact overlap with the other factors.

The idea that wheat was involved in schizophrenia originated from Dr F. Curtis Dohan, a psychiatrist working at the University of Pennsylvania hospital in Philadelphia. Studying the official medical statistics for schizophrenia from many countries, he noticed that there had been a marked fall in the number of cases of schizophrenia in countries where there had been food shortages and rationing during the Second World War. After the war the incidence of schizophrenia had returned to its former level. The most significant change in the national diet of these countries during the war had been a drop in the consumption of wheat products. Schizophrenia, he knew, tended to be more common in countries where the staple diet was based on wheat, corn, or rye. So he wondered whether a cereal-free diet might help his schizophrenic patients.

He put his theory to the test by dividing his schizophrenic patients into two groups, one of which was given a cereal-free diet and the other a normal hospital diet replete with cereal products. The patients who were deprived of cereals did indeed do much better; their symptoms receded and some who had been institutionalized for years were discharged and allowed to go home or even back to work.

Dr Dohan's report, published in a Scandinavian psychiatric journal in 1966, roused little but scepticism from his professional colleagues. They pointed out that schizophrenics always tend to get better if they have a lot of attention paid to them, especially if they have been isolated in a hospital for years. The diet, they suggested, was no more than an elaborate placebo.

Undaunted, Dohan then proceeded to study coeliac disease, which was undeniably associated with cereal allergy. He found that coeliac disease was much commoner among schizophrenics than in the general population. Admittedly only one in a hundred schizophrenics also had coeliac disease, but this was still a much higher incidence than normal.

Nevertheless, his idea of a link between wheat and schizophrenia was so out of line with contemporary thought that no one felt it would be worthwhile sticking out his professional neck by testing the method for himself. It was not until ten years after Dohan had published his paper that his findings were corroborated by two other psychiatrists, Drs M. M. Singh and S. R. Kay. Writing in the journal *Science*, they reported that some of their patients had responded well to a cereal-free and milk-free diet and that this improvement apparently could not be attributed to any other change in their therapy or environment.

If wheat allergy is a cause of schizophrenia, it would be interesting to know why this allergy affects the brain rather than the gut or any other part of the body. The answer to this question may be provided by those 'natural opiates', the endorphins.

Discovered only a few years ago by researchers at Aberdeen University, the endorphins are substances produced by the pituitary gland when the body is subjected to painful stimuli. The scientists who discovered their existence, Dr John Hughes and Professor Hans Kosterlitz, were specialists in drug addiction. They knew that opiate drugs like morphine and heroin attached themselves to a particular kind of receptor in the brain. These receptors posed an interesting question: had they just been designed to bind a foreign chemical distilled from poppies — or were they really intended for some substance produced by the body? They eventually found that there were indeed natural substances which were attracted to the same receptors as morphine and heroin. They also had a similar effect to these drugs — they could relieve pain, and they were addictive.

Drug companies have not yet been able to produce a synthetic endorphin which relieves pain and is not addictive. However, endorphins have produced an explanation for the pain relief which can be produced by acupuncture needles and electrical stimulation. A needle twirled in the skin or a light electric current will both stimulate the body to produce endorphins. Exactly how this happens we do not know, but both these forms of treatment cause a significant increase in the amount of endorphin in the spinal fluid.

Endorphins were described in a recent BBC TV programme as 'the keys to paradise'. In truth they may also be the keys to hell. Large amounts of endorphin given to animals have caused catatonia. And unusually high levels of endorphins have been found in the spinal fluid of people suffering from schizophrenia.

One way to explain this excess of endorphin would be to identify a defective mechanism in the body's metabolism, but no one has yet been able to do this. What does now seem likely is that these endorphins are coming from outside the body.

Endorphins are peptides, chains of amino acids. Proteins are complex peptide structures which can be broken down by enzymes into smaller peptides. Many of the proteins in food contain peptide complexes which are similar to endorphins. In other words, it is theoretically possible for food proteins to be broken down into substances which will have an effect on the central nervous system. This may sound far-fetched, but recent research has shown that this does in fact happen when gluten is broken down in the stomach.

Dr W. A. Klee and his colleagues at the National Institute of Mental Health Research in the United States have found that partially digested gluten can act in exactly the same way as opiate drugs or endorphins. To distinguish these broken-down products from endorphins, which are by definition substances produced in the body, Dr Klee calls them 'exorphins' — which is a Greek way of saying 'morphine-like substances coming from outside the body'.

In a healthy, efficient stomach these exorphins would probably be broken down by enzymes into smaller harmless peptides. But Dr Klee's research team has demonstrated that this does not always happen, and that exorphins can sometimes pass through the lining of the gut into the blood-stream. In fact they might not even have to get into the blood-stream and be carried to the brain to do their damage. For some reason understood by the Almighty alone, the gut is full of those receptors which attract endorphins and morphine. We can only speculate whether exorphins are triggering mental reactions by latching on to receptors in the gut, but the idea of food causing mental disease certainly looks much less ridiculous now than when it was first put forward.

Coeliac disease is not the only gastrointestinal disorder which has been linked with schizophrenia. Professors V. M. and G. A. Buscaino of Naples have looked for gut diseases in several hundred schizophrenics; they diagnosed abnormal liver function in 83 per cent; gastric inflammation in 50 per cent; gastroenteritis in 88 per cent; and colitis in 92 per cent. Kidney disease is also commoner in schizophrenics than in the general population. Disorders of the gut, liver and kidney can allow all manner of toxic substances to enter and pass unchecked through the blood-stream, and it now seems highly likely that these toxins can aggravate, if not cause, schizophrenia.

The first clue that schizophrenia could result from a kind of poisoning came from schizophrenic patients who were being treated for kidney disease on renal dialysis units. These units, better known as kidney machines, take the place of the patient's useless kidneys by filtering waste products out of the blood. They do not cure the disease, and each patient has to undergo regular dialysis to remove the constant accumulation of dead cells, salts and other useless breakdown products. When schizophrenics with kidney failure were first put into kidney machines, it became apparent that their mental symptoms were clearing up too.

Since then, doctors in the United States and Britain have tried dialysis on schizophrenics without obvious kidney disease and have found that many of them get better too. For instance, out of a group of fourteen schizophrenics dialysed by the American doctors Cade and Wagemaker, nine were judged to be greatly improved, two experienced a moderate improvement and three did not appear to benefit. Dialysis is not yet widely used on schizophrenics who do not have kidney disease, but there are a number of clinical trials being conducted into this treatment.

If schizophrenics do benefit from dialysis, we can only assume that it is the result of harmful substances being taken out of their system. Many potential poisons are removed by dialysis, but one substance which has so far only been found in schizophrenic patients' dialysis extracts seems particularly relevant to the subject in hand: it is an abnormal endorphin.

This endorphin — leucine endorphin, to give it its full name — was found by a University of California research team who were analysing the dialysis extracts from Dr Cade and Dr Wagemaker's schizophrenic patients. As yet no one can be sure where this endorphin came from in the first place. Was it produced naturally in the brain, or was it a partially broken-down food protein?

If breakdown products from semi-digested wheat are similar to the natural opiates, we have an explanation for the addiction which clinical ecologists claim to be a result of food allergy. The food could be acting just like morphine or heroin acts on a drug addict, latching onto the same receptors and stimulating the same areas of the central nervous system. This would also explain why food addicts get unpleasant withdrawal symptoms when they first go on an exclusion diet and stop taking the food which is causing their problems. Healthy people do not become addicted to their endorphins because these substances are released in tiny quantities and are quickly broken down by enzymes. We can become addicted to heroin and morphine because our bodies do not have a well-developed enzyme system for breaking these drugs down. But animal experiments have proved that it is possible to become addicted to endorphins if they are continuously pumped into the body by artifical means. Is this very different from feeding wheat into the stomach of someone who is unable to break the proteins down properly and is therefore constantly overloading himself with exorphins? Speculative perhaps, but quite possible.

Exorphins suggest that schizophrenia may be a kind of food poisoning which only affects people with faulty digestion. But there are other ways wheat could cause brain damage. In May 1978 Drs David Freed and Barry Durrant told readers of the *British Medical Journal* that they had found abnormally high amounts of antibody to wheat and several other foods in the blood of people suffering from schizophrenia, dementia and other mental disorders. They have since repeated these investigations on schizophrenic patients and confirmed that antibodies to wheat and, to a lesser extent, rye are unusually common in these people. Obviously the presence of antibodies does not prove that the foods are the cause of the schizophrenia, but it does offer further circumstantial evidence linking mental disease with food allergy.

This opinion is backed by Dr W. A. Hemmings, an immunologist at the University College of North Wales, well known in scientific circles for his research into the way proteins cross tissue membranes. In the *Lancet* in March 1978 he commented that food allergy, especially wheat allergy, was a very likely cause of mental symptoms:

Large amounts of high molecular weight breakdown products (BDP) of dietary protein pass through the gut wall . . . . Much of the BDP retains its original antigenicity when in the tissue after digestion and passage through the circulation, and direct reactions with cellular antibody are thus possible. The enormous variety of protein structures which must arise from partial cleavage of dietary proteins may produce pharmacological and toxicological effects. Among the peptic degradation products of alpha-gliadin, one polypeptide had endorphine-like activity . . . . Psychological symptoms are not unexpected since BDP appear to pass the blood/brain barrier. These fragments may be directly cytotoxic [poisonous] to neural [brain] cells, have subtle pharmacological actions, or trigger a cerebral allergic reaction if antibody of the appropriate class is also present in the brain.

Dr Hemmings' research has also shown that proteins, their breakdown products and antibodies from cow's milk can pass into mother's milk and can even cross the placenta and get into the unborn foetus. In this way a baby could be poisoned or sensitized to a food before it is born or when its immune system is only poorly developed.

Even if we assume that food allergy is involved in schizophrenia, there is still a great deal to be explained. Why, for instance, does the disease not come on until late adolescence? Like heart disease and cancer, schizophrenia very possibly results from a combination of factors, some of which are inherited and some of which can be found in the environment. Food allergy may turn out to be a factor in only a small minority of cases, but when we consider that half a million Britons and over two million Americans now living will suffer from this disease at some time during their lives, this 'small' minority may still number in the tens of thousands of miserable people.

10
Obesity and Alcoholism

Height: five feet nothing? Weight: two hundred pounds? Do you raid the kitchen at night and eat half a box of cornflakes at one sitting? If you open a packet of biscuits, do they disappear in ten minutes flat — into your mouth?

If the answer to the above question is 'yes', you're not just fat, you're addicted. And you probably don't need me to tell you so.

Compulsive eating is not only a habit of fat people. Plenty of 'normal' or even skinny people like to binge on foods like chocolate and biscuits. The reason they do not get very fat probably lies in their metabolism: some people just expend more energy than others and are therefore less likely to put on weight. But whether they are fat or thin, compulsive eaters almost invariably go for sweet or starchy foods. Few are tempted to glut themselves on carrots or kippers or any meat, fruit or vegetable. If they go for sandwiches or hamburgers, they are more interested in the bread or bun than what lies in the middle.

Compulsive eating is usually attributed to 'emotional problems', often with a Freudian tag suggesting that the eater has an unrequited need for 'oral gratification'. This explanation has yielded little in the way of useful suggestions for treating obesity. The amphetamine drugs do put you in a lively mood, but — like almost all the drugs used to suppress appetite — they lose their effect quite quickly. They are also dangerous, because they lead to dependence, an inclination to take ever greater doses to maintain the 'high', and in the end to mental breakdown.

In 1975 the Department of Health sent out a boldly worded circular to all British family doctors, pointing out that appetite-suppressant drugs were costing the country £2.5 million a year (at 1973 prices) and suggesting that they probably did very little good. Quoting the standard drug reference book used by doctors, *The British National Formulary,* the circular proclaimed that 'Appetite-suppressant drugs have little place in the management of the obese patient and there is no substitute for willpower.'

The department's advice was a little harsh and doubtless based more on its concern about the national drug bill than any practical consideration about how the doctor should set about encouraging his fat patients to lose weight. These drugs, used in moderation at the beginning of a weight-reduction course, can at least show fat people that it is possible to lose weight by eating less.

Starchy sugary foods are high in calories and are therefore more likely to make you fat than an equivalent volume of carrots. But few researchers have addressed themselves to the question 'Why do compulsive eaters go for these refined carbohydrates?'

Dr Ted Randolph in the United States and Dr Richard Mackarness in Britain believe that compulsive eating is an addiction which develops from an allergy. According to their stress theory of allergy which I outlined in Chapter 2, an allergic person who continues to eat an allergenic food will adapt her or himself to the stress the allergic reactions impose on the system. This process of adaptation taxes the body's hormonal resources and brings about a change in body chemistry which the sufferer comes to regard as normal. If the food is withdrawn from the diet, its absence will begin to make the body chemistry revert to its original state, but the patient will experience this as disagreeable withdrawal symptoms and immediately crave the food which will put him back into the stressed condition which he regarded as 'normal' and desirable. In this way the person becomes hooked on a food and can only become unhooked if it is left out of the diet for at least several days.

Now, although not everyone would agree with this theory about stress, there is other good evidence to support the idea of food addiction. Several food allergists have reported that ingestion of a food allergen, especially wheat or other cereals, is followed by a bout of hypoglycaemia, a fall in blood sugar levels. Dr Len McEwen of St Mary's Hospital, London, told me that this reaction invariably happens in his mentally disturbed patients who are allergic to wheat.

And Dr J. C. Breneman in his textbook *Basics of Food Allergy* comments that 'Hypoglycaemia is a frequent laboratory and clinical finding produced by ingestion of food allergens. It appears within two to six hours and the symptoms include light-headedness, flushing, confusion, sweaty, weak sensations and even fainting spells or convulsions'. Why this hypoglycaemia should occur, no one knows, but its effect is to make the sufferer crave something sweet which will return blood sugar levels to normal. Obesity, Dr Breneman claims, is often the result of this recurring urge to top up with carbohydrate.

The other piece of evidence which supports the idea of food addiction takes us back to our old friends the endorphins. In 1978 a team of scientists and psychologists from Temple University, Philadelphia, and the US National Institue of Mental Health reported in *Science* that fat rats and mice produced much more endorphin than thin rats and mice. The fat animals had been specially bred through several generations from rats and mice which had a genetic tendency to be fat. When they were given a dose of naloxone, the drug which counteracts morphine and endorphins, they stopped eating as much as they had before. The drug has no effect on the thin mice and rats, who carried on eating as normal.

The implication of this study is that obese creatures may be addicted to their endorphins just as heroin and morphine addicts are addicted to their drugs. Compulsive eaters and narcotic addicts experience similar withdrawal symptoms and also tend to relapse into their old addictive habits at the least temptation.

Why do the animals produce so much endorphin? we might ask. There are several possible explanations, all of them speculative. It could be a stress reaction: when an animal is under stress its pituitary gland is stimulated to release the hormone which sets the adrenal glands in action. At the same time it also releases endorphins. This explains why soldiers in the heat of battle do not feel their wounds; the painful stimuli are blocked by endorphins. If an allergic person was in a permanent state of stress he would be constantly producing endorphins, and could, theoretically at least, get hooked on them.

Alternatively, could these addictive substances be exorphins rather than endorphins? Do these carefully bred fat rats have a congenital inability to break down food proteins well enough to prevent potent peptides attaching themselves to the many endorphin receptors in the gut or pushing through into the bloodstream? Rodent diets are of course full of cereals, which we know to be the source of exorphins.

Both these ideas are based on the assumption that the animals were unable to tolerate foods as well as their genetically normal thin cousins. Compulsive eating can therefore be regarded as the result of an allergy.

The hypoglycaemia which results from eating wheat could explain why some people with food allergy have been diagnosed as epileptic. A fall in blood sugar makes you hungry, but it also causes a number of mental reactions, beginning with uneasiness and a feeling of drunkenness, and proceeding — if the blood sugar level falls very low — to unconsciousness or fits.

Wheat is not the only food to have been associated with fits, however. Dr Breneman reports from his own clinical experience that 'approximately fifteen per cent of grand mal epileptic patients can trigger their grand mal seizures by the ingestion of known food allergens. Milk is the most common offender, although almost any food might be incriminated.'

A little five-year-old girl who was treated by the Massachusetts psychiatrist Dr William Philpott illustrates how fits can be brought on by many foods. She had been suffering as many as twenty seizures a day, and drugs had only provided her with mild relief. But when she was taken off her drugs and fasted for a few days, her fits disappeared. Individual foods were then introduced into her diet one by one. Some foods caused no problems, but twelve items were promptly followed by convulsions. Once these foods were permanently removed from her diet, she was only rarely troubled by her epilepsy and was able to come off her previous medication.

The little girl's blood sugar levels were apparently not recorded, but it is of course quite conceivable that her fits were not being caused by hypoglycaemia. We know that allergies can cause inflammation in almost any part of the body which has been sensitized; it is therefore reasonable to suggest that allergic people may get a rash or swelling in the brain itself. We know from Dr Hemmings' work that food particles can be carried into the brain via the blood-stream, so there is a distinct possibility that allergic people could suffer all manner of mental symptoms resulting from an inflammation of part of the brain.

This little digression into epilepsy and mental disorders has taken us away from the subject of obesity and addiction, but it does show, I hope, how diverse food reactions can be both in their mechanism and effect.

If a compulsive eater is addicted to cereal foods, the only useful advice he can be offered is: give them up. A number of doctors have suggested diets which make this abstinence more acceptable. Richard Mackarness in England, Blake Donaldson and the late Alfred Pennington in the United States and Ray Lawson of Canada have all reported remarkable success with diets which eliminate all cereals but which allow you to eat as much meat as you like. Drs Lawson and Donaldson base their ideas on studies of Eskimo peoples who eat vast quantities of fatty meat but very few fresh vegetables and almost no cereals and who appear to suffer few of the 'diseases of civilization' such as obesity, heart disease and dental caries. Mackarness calls his high-meat, high-fat diet a 'Stone Age diet' because it corresponds with the diet man used to eat before he took up growing crops for food. High-fat diets are extremely unfashionable with the majority of the medical profession today because statistical evidence shows that a high intake of animal fats from meat and milk is associated with heart disease. Nor does everyone lose weight by going on these diets; in a survey of slimming methods conducted by the Consumers' Association some people reported that they had put on weight by following a Stone Age diet even though they had followed the dietary instructions to the letter. In the diet's favour, it should be said that most people on a high-fat, high-meat diet do not feel as hungry as those who go on the more conventional low-fat, low-carbohydrate diets.

Dr Randolph believes that alcoholism, like obesity, can be the result of a food allergy. But he points out that the originator of this idea was the psychiatrist Francis Hare, who practised in Australia and later in England in the early part of this century. Dr Hare's first book,

The Food Factor in Disease, was published in 1906 and though it seems to have aroused little interest at the time, its observations and theories were in many ways similar to those of modern clinical ecologists. He declared that migraine, asthma, bronchitis, eczema, stomach troubles, angina, high blood-pressure, gout, arthritis and several degenerative diseases were caused by excessive consumption of 'carbonaceous' or carbohydrate foods, particularly those containing refined sugar, starch and alcohol. He found that many of his patients got better when these foods were restricted and replaced with protein-rich foods, and he came to the conclusion that some people had difficulty in metabolizing carbohydrates.

In 1912 he published his second book, *On Alcoholism,* which was based on his experiences as medical director of the Norwood Sanitarium, an asylum in Beckenham, Kent. He noticed that the alcoholic's craving for drink followed a pattern quite like the carbohydrate addict's craving for sweet or starchy foods. There were certain periods of the day when the craving was most marked: in food addicts this was often late at night, and in alcoholics it was early in the morning, an hour or so before lunch and, worst of all, in the early evening before dinner.

He also pointed out that alcoholism killed the desire for sweet foods, but that a 'sweet tooth' almost always returned after the alcoholic had given up drinking. This return of the desire for sweets was very often accompanied by an outbreak of typical allgeric symptoms like rashes or asthma. He noticed that many of his patients suffering from depression and other mental illnesses had a similar fluctuation in their symptoms: if their mental symptoms remitted for a while, they would be replaced by skin eruptions and/or respiratory complaints. Interestingly, these observations coincided with those made by another English psychiatrist, George Savage, some thirty years earlier.

Dr Hare wrote this book at a time when alcoholism was still widely believed to be a moral rather than a medical problem and when the word allergy had barely been invented, let alone understood. Though Hare had not used the terms allergy and addiction, Randolph, reading his books some forty years later, recognized in Hare's descriptions the same phenomena that he was seeing in his own food-allergic patients.

As I mentioned briefly in Chapter 3, Randolph had first become interested in alcoholism when he noticed that his patients reacted as strongly to spirits distilled from food as they did to the food itself. If grape-sensitive patients drank wine or if corn-sensitive patients drank corn liquors they would become groggy and sick after taking a very small amount, though they appeared to have a normal tolerance of alcoholic beverages brewed from foods to which they were not allergic.

Studying alcoholic patients, Randolph came to the conclusion that they were addicted not so such to alcohol as to the grain or fruit from which their favourite tipple was derived. Using the provocation tests devised for diagnosing food allergy, he examined a group of alcoholics who had recently 'gone on the wagon', and found that those who did not display an untoward reaction to corn or grape would not react badly to corn or grape spirits either. He reasoned that alcoholism was like the kind of 'masked allergy' described by his colleague Herbert Rinkel: the first time you drank a liquor made from a food to which you were allergic you felt sick, and you would continue to feel sick if you continued to take it only now and then. But if, like Rinkel and his eggs, you took it very regularly, your system would adapt to it until you reached the point where a brief abstinence would cause unpleasant withdrawal symptoms which could only be eradicated by taking another drink.

Randolph wrote up his theory and sent the paper off to the editor of a medical journal specializing in studies on alcoholism. The editor of the journal had expressed interest in his work and had been the first to suggest that it should be published. But when he got the finished paper he began to have second thoughts. Randolph's theory was so out of line with contemporary thinking that he wondered whether it was very sound. The paper sat on his desk for two years and would probably have been sitting there still had Randolph not called him one day to ask what had become of it. Eventually the editor was persuaded to send it off to another specialist to be vetted. As luck would have it, the doctor he chose was an old colleague of Randolph's, who was only too willing to put in a good word. So the paper finally did get published in 1956.

Publication is only the first step in getting a theory accepted. The next stage is to put it into practice, and in this Dr Randolph had only had partial success. He found that a few of the acoholics he treated could overcome their problem without having to give drink up altogether, but only if they stayed off beverages made from foods to which they were allergic, and only drank in moderation. The difficulties were compounded by the fact that very few drinks contained alcohol from a single source. Nearly all drinks also had corn or beet sugar added to them. And most alcohol still contains traces of yeast, a quite common allergen. Dr Randolph's liberal approach to alcoholism does not insist on total abstinence from drink, and this has not endeared him to Alcoholics Anonymous, the principal organization which helps alcoholics, and which has complete abstinence as its basic rule.

All things considered then, the food addiction theory to alcoholism may be interesting, but it is hard to put into practice to help really hard drinkers. In fact anyone with food allergy is probably best advised to be very wary of alcohol, whatever its source. Alcohol aggravates reactions to allergenic foods and it can also bring out reactions which would not necessarily occur if the food was taken alone. Some people can eat shrimp, for instance, but will get an acute reaction — swelling, rash or diarrhoea — if they are drinking alcohol at the same time. Champagne quite often makes asthmatics suffer, and migraine sufferers often get their headaches after drinking, especially Italian red wine.

The link between red wine and migraine may have less to do with alcohol than with the presence of the amino acid tyramine, which is also found in chocolate, cheese, pickled herring, broad beans and onions. Some people who suffer from migraine are short of an enzyme called monoamine oxidase, which breaks down tyramine. If too much tyramine builds up in the blood, it sets off a chemical chain reaction which causes blood vessels in the head to contract.

Beers particularly should be regarded with as much mistrust as any highly processed food. In 1978 the British Ministry of Agriculture's Food Additives and Contaminants Committee listed more than sixty additives used in the production of beer or as preservatives. The names of some of these substances are probably more terrifying than their toxic or allergic potential. The soberest of judges would have difficulty with polyvinylpolypyrrolidone, which is added to stop beer going cloudy. And how about dimethylpolysiloxane, which is added to prevent beer from foaming too much? Try pronouncing that one the next time you are slumped over the saloon bar.

Although most of these chemicals were, in the words of *The Times*, 'given a clean bill of health' by the committee (this is always an ominous statement, which should be taken to imply that the risks to life are less important than the risks to commerce or government if the substance is withdrawn), some additives were withdrawn for further toxicological studies. Among these were certain enzyme preparations which enabled brewers to use barley rather than malt, which is rather more expensive, to manufacture their products.

Additives, combined with the fact that brewers are very secretive about their recipes, make it very hard for a drinker to know what the liquid in his glass actually consists of. Liverpool physician Dr Ronald Finn was once confronted by a patient who was obviously allergic to one of the ingredients of his favourite stout. The man was a docker, who drank no more than his mates but who had recently started turning bright red, just like the setting sun, whenever he drank more than a pint.

His fellow drinkers thought it was a great joke and told him that he was indulging a bit more than he should. This strange rubicund affliction and the taunts of his friends were making him apprehensive about going into the pub, which until then had been the cornerstone of his social life. Having ascertained that the man was not drinking heavily and that his red face was not just the effect of alcohol alone, the doctor suggested that he should try drinking other beers to see if they made him blush too. Some did, others had less of an effect, and finally the docker found a light ale which he could drink without any risk of jeopardizing his complexion. 'He was one of my most grateful patients', Dr Finn told me.

11
Arthritis

Arthritis and rheumatism are blanket terms which cover a variety of muscle and joint disorders. The commonest of these chronic diseases are osteoarthrosis (often called osteoarthritis), rheumatoid arthritis and gout. Osteoarthrosis is a degeneration of the smooth cartilage in joints, especially the weight-bearing joints in the legs and spine. Once this cartilage goes, the bones in the joint rub together, causing pain and restricted movement. Gout is an inflammation of joints, often the big toe joint; its principal characteristic is a build-up of uric acid crystals in tissues around the joint. Rheumatoid arthritis is basically a disease of the connective tissue around joints, especially in the hands and fingers. The joint becomes inflamed, and this often triggers a severe muscle spasm which can in time deform or dislocate the joint almost irreparably.

The causes of these diseases are not really understood. Osteoarthrosis is often said to be the result of wear and tear, but recent research has shown that osteoarthrosed joints contain precipitates of tiny crystals rather like those found in gout. These crystals are just as likely a cause as wear and tear, though it is a mystery how they get there. Gout was believed to be caused by eating foods like liver, kidney and peas which are rich in uric acid, but elimination of such foods has negligible benefits. Gout could result from overproduction of uric acid or defective excretion. Rheumatoid arthritis is the greatest puzzle. The most popular current explanation is that it is an autoimmune disease, in which the patient develops antibodies to his own tissues. Antibodies to certain cells are found in rheumatoid patients, and it is possible that these antibodies are formed when cells are attacked by a virus. The immune system recognizes these virally infected cells as abnormal and makes antibody to elimate them. The antibody is only partially successful in its attempts to get rid of the cells, and immune complexes are formed (see Appendix I) which cause inflammation.

That, very briefly, is the conventional modern immunological concept of rheumatoid arthritis. Autoimmunity is a form of allergy, but immunologists tend to look into the body in their search for the causes of the disease rather than look outside for possible environmental factors. This approach has brought us nowhere near a cure. The principal treatments for rheumatoid arthritis are anti-inflammatory drugs like indomethacin, which control pain and inflammation, or steroids, which are very effective at reducing inflammation, but whose adverse effects make them only suitable for severe advanced cases. Neither form of drug therapy eradicates the underlying disease process.

Although not many specialists have looked for environmental causes, they are almost certainly a critical factor. Bantu people, for example, who live on rural reservations in South Africa, rarely suffer from rheumatoid arthritis, but they do get the disease as commonly as white people once they move to the cities. It would seem that something in the city air or in their changed diet must be responsible.

Many clinical ecologists have claimed that patients suffering from rheumatic and arthritic diseases have improved considerably after eliminating foods to which they were apparently allergic, and have got their symptoms back when they ate these foods again. Let us look at a few cases.

A thirty-five-year-old registered nurse, who since her childhood had suffered from recurrent sinus trouble, diarrhoea and indigestion, got inflamed tendons in her wrists a few months after moving into a new home in 1969. This inflammation spread quickly, and was soon affecting her right shoulder and knee, and after about a year it had progressed into her hands and feet and her other shoulder and knee. Her old sinus trouble cleared up during these bouts of arthritis, but tended to recur when the inflammation subsided. Just before the arthritic spells began, she would invariably feel irritable, tired and depressed.

By 1972 her arthritis was so bad that she was admitted to a

hospital to have the inflamed synovial membrane in her right knee joint surgically removed. The operation did not do a great deal of good, and by now her left knee was as incapacitated as the right knee had been. She then sought treatment from a hospital running an environmental control programme, which involved a five-day fast, followed by a gradual exposure to single foods and chemicals.

After a five-day fast she was able to walk without crutches and her inflammation had subsided noticeably. She did not react badly to organically grown, uncontaminated foods, but commercial forms of corn, cane, apple, lamb, orange, grape, egg, wheat, pork, rice, lobster tail and beef all brought on arthritic pain. The pains came less than fifteen minutes after eating corn or cane, about three hours after beef and lobster. Reactions to the other foods were felt within the hour. She was able to drink pure tomato juice, but she got stiff joints, fatigue, irritability and depression after drinking tomato juice which came from a can. The doctor was able to reverse all these adverse reactions by giving her a dose of bicarbonate of soda in water.

When she was discharged she was advised to avoid foods which were possibly chemically contaminated and to drink only unchlorinated water. By so doing she has steadily improved and only has attacks of arthritic pain when she inadvertently eats chemically tainted foods.

It is perhaps significant that this lady had a history of allergy. It seems that almost everyone with arthritis who has responded well to ecological treatment had previously suffered from rhinitis, asthmas, asthma, eczema or some other typically allergic complaint.

A nine-year-old schoolgirl, who used to get skin rashes after eating oranges, developed arthritis in her ankles and knees, and eventually had to have a synovectomy of her right knee. Subsequently, in 1973 she was taken into an environmental unit. After the first two days of fasting she suffered from nausea and headaches, but at the end of four days these had gone and her joints were more mobile and less painful than they had been for months. Feeding tests then began, and she suffered joint pains, muscle cramps and feelings of irritability and depression a few hours after eating wheat, yeast, milk, rice and beef. When she went back home, she improved and remained well on a diet which excluded these foods. She had a flare-up of her arthritis in the autumn when the gas-fired central heating was turned on. Her family then moved to an electrically equipped house, since when she has been symptom-free, except for a little pain and a click in her synovectomized knee, for which she has had physiotherapy. She has given up all drugs.

A seventy-eight-year-old retired businessman had suffered from perennial rhinitis for about thirty years and during the previous eight years had had occasional attacks of arthritis in his hands. Not long before he was admitted to the environmental unit this arthritis had got much worse and had spread to his right elbow, shoulders, knees and right hip. By the time he was admitted to the unit his hands were so swollen that he could barely pick up a knife and fork to eat, and he refused to shake hands.

After the five-day fast the pain in all his joints had subsided, though his hands were still rather swollen. Food tests for corn were followed by nausea and diarrhoea after three hours and by joint pains after six hours. Just over three hours after eating wheat, his eyes and nose began to run, though this subsided after a short time. He awoke with joint pain thirteen hours after being fed beets and beet sugar. No other food, organic or commercial, was followed by pain or inflammation.

When he was discharged from the unit he was free of symptoms. Eight months later he tried reintroducing wheat into his diet, and this produced no bad effect until he started eating wheat products twice a day and also added corn and beet sugar to his diet. The swelling and pain subsided when he dropped these items, and he was still symptom-free four years later.

These are three out of two hundred cases of arthritis treated by Dr Ted Randolph and his colleagues in the environmental unit in a hospital just outside Chicago. Not all responded so well, and a few were dismal failures. He has kept detailed records of these cases to answer his critics who laughed him to scorn when he first suggested that food and chemical allergy might play a part in arthritic disease.

Dr Randolph is not the only doctor who has had such success. In 1978 Dr F. Murray Carroll of North Carolina reported the results of a three-and-a-half-year-long study he had made of arthritic patients. He also found that most of his patients had had a past history of allergic complaints like asthma, migraine and gastro-intestinal disorders.

During those three and a half years he brought over three hundred arthritic patients into the hospital for a fast followed by food testing. The patients were challenged with about forty foods each. Those which most commonly provoked symptoms were corn (37 per cent), wheat (27 per cent), milk (23 per cent), coffee (22 per cent), tea (22 per cent), sugar (20 per cent), pork (19 per cent), apples (14 per cent), cola drinks (14 per cent), oranges (12 per cent), chocolate (11 per cent), beef (9 per cent), tomatoes (9 per cent), butter beans (9 per cent) and peanuts (8 per cent).

After being discharged, the patients were all asked to fill in a questionnaire saying how and whether they had benefited from their hospital stay. Only 44 per cent of the 316 patients bothered to return their quesionnaires, so it is difficult to get an exact idea of the number who did benefit. But from the replies he did receive it seems that the vast majority of those who felt inclined to fill in the questionnaire had done very well.

The idea is to keep exposure to potential allergens to a minimum. And many food allergists believe that by following such a diet you can lose an allergy to a food which previously caused problems when eaten regularly in large amounts. What Dr Carroll wanted to know was whether the benefits of the hospital treatment could be kept up afterwards by following a rotary diet. In this kind of diet you take care not to eat particular foods more than once or twice every few days. One of the best ways to assess the merits of a rotary diet was to see whether his arthritic patients could give up or reduce the amount of pain-killing drugs they were taking. So the next part of the questionnaire asked patients to say whether they had followed a rotary diet or not and how they had fared. Table VII shows their replies.

From this we see that most of the patients had been able to reduce

their consumption of pain-killers to a certain extent. But those who
followed the rotary diet seemed to do a lot better than those who
did not.

Ninety-eight per cent of those with osteoarthritis and 91 per cent
of those with rheumatoid arthritis said that their condition had
improved while they were in the hospital, and nearly all of them
said that the improvement had resulted from eliminating the
allergenic foods. 'Improvement' does of course have a broad
meaning, and could range from mild relief of pain and swelling
to complete remission. But when Dr Carroll asked those who said
they had improved to assess how much they had improved in terms
of pain relief, reduction of swelling and general mobility, 27 per
cent of the osteoarthritics and 11 per cent of the rheumatoids said
they were 100 per cent better, and about half of each group said
that they were somewhere between 50 per cent and completely
better after avoiding allergenic foods.

Table VII Replies to Dr Carroll's questionnaire

		Given up all drugs %	Reduced drugs by more than 70 per cent %	Reduced drugs by less than 70 per cent %
Osteoarthritic patients	Following rotary diet	57	6	15
	Not following rotary diet	37	7	37
Rheumatoid patients	Following rotary diet	59	19	11
	Not following rotary diet	10	10	70

(Note: If you add up each row of figures they might not come to 100 per cent; this is because
some patients either had not been prescribed drugs before or were not able to give a
clear answer.)

We have to remember that rather less than half of his patients
had bothered to respond to his questionnaire. But even if we assume
that those who did not reply had not benefited at all, the success

rate was still very high for a therapy which many of his medical colleagues would have scorned as quackery.

These statistics and case histories offer evidence that food allergy plays more than a small part in arthritis. Chemical allergy may play a part too. It is hard to explain why an allergy should manifest itself in the joints, but we have already seen how diverse the effects of allergy can be and how many toxicological, pharmacological and immunological reactions can be caused by the breakdown of food in the body. The main point is that fasting and elimination diets can help some sufferers, and as well as being effective, they are cheap and safe.

12

Healthy and Not So Healthy Food

In the last few chapters we have seen how common and chronic diseases can be caused or aggravated by foods and chemicals. It seems that allergy — in the widest sense of the word — is responsible, in part or in whole, for an enormous range of illnesses which are generally believed to have nothing in common with each other. If you asked most doctors to say what connection there was between arthritis and migraine, or between asthma and duodenal ulcers, they would think you were ignorant, cranky or crazy. But it is clear that common foods do have something to do with these various afflictions, and that many people can get better by altering their diet.

During the past century the medical profession has become more and more specialized. Doctors who want to make a career for themselves have been obliged to concentrate on particular diseases in particular parts of the body just to be able to keep up with the mass of research and modern therapeutic techniques. But although this super-specialization has brought some real breakthroughs in the understanding and treatment of disease, the people of the Western world are not living any longer, nor are they noticeably healthier than they were fifty years ago. Some diseases — tuberculosis, for example — have almost disappeared, but others — such as obesity, cancer and mental illness — are still on the increase.

The conventional medical approach to disease is to take a sick person and see what is the matter with him or her. But we have seen that a great deal of illness is not the result of a fault in the patient but is due more to a fault in their diet or environment. Heredity does seem to make some people more vulnerable to allergy than others, but the disease they suffer is brought on by exposure — in the womb, at the breast or bottle, at the table or in the polluted air — to food or chemicals. In the normal course of events someone with migraine would be referred to a neurologist, someone with schizophrenia to a psychiatrist, someone with skin disease to a dermatologist, someone with arthritis to a rheumatologist, and so on. But if a substantial proportion of these people are really the victims of their environment, wouldn't it make more sense for them first to seek the help of an ecologist? At present, this cannot be done, because there are just not enough medical ecologists to go around. Nor are they all trusted by their colleagues.

Recent years have also seen a growing mistrust of the medical profession on the part of the general public. People are less inclined to take their doctor's word for gospel and are increasingly turning to alternative practitioners and philosophers for advice on healthy living. A landmark in this antimedical movement was the publication in 1975 of Ivan Illich's book *Medical Nemesis,* in which the author, a Jesuit teacher and political philosopher, declared that 'The medical establishment has become a major threat to health'. I suspect that much of Illich's dislike of the medical profession is derived from his jealousy, as a Catholic, of doctors who have largely taken over the Church's traditional role as confessors and providers of hope to the people. Nevertheless, his discontent with modern medicine has been echoed by some doctors like Professor Thomas McKeown, who, in his book *The Role of Medicine: Dream Mirage or Nemesis?,* suggested that 'medical intervention has made and can be expected to make a relatively small contribution to the prevention of sickness and death'.

As far as diet and health are concerned, there has been no shortage of theorists prepared to exploit (both in the good and bad senses of that word) the rift between the public and conventional medical science. Vegans, vegetarians, 'fruitarians', propagandists for macrobiotics and other dietary regimes have attracted sympathetic interest from people who twenty years ago would have dismissed such things as silly fads. So just in case any readers have been put off their normal diet by this book that they are considering one of these alternatives, I would like to outline very briefly their virtues and vices.

Vegans and vegetarians both avoid eating meat and fish, and vegans are also obliged to refuse eggs and milk. Their diets generally result in their consuming fewer calories than people on a normal omnivorous diet, and they therefore tend to be slimmer than omnivores. This is a strong point in their favour. It does seem, however, that a healthy diet needs to be diverse. The deficiencies in vitamins, essential amino acids and the trace elements which affect some vegetarians and vegans are very often due to their eating a narrow diet. No plant contains all the necessary ingredients for making the human body function at full efficiency.

Proteins are the building blocks of living matter; they are chains of amino acids, which, when eaten, are taken apart and reconstructed into the particular patterns of human tissue. It hardly matters whether proteins come from meat or plants; what does matter is that they contain the right proportion of raw material in the form of amino acids for the construction of new cells. Vitamins are substances which the body needs to accomplish certain functions, but which it cannot make itself by rearranging proteins. Vitamins therefore have to be provided ready-made via the diet.

Except for soya beans, plant foods generally lack some of the essential amino acids. A diet based on cereals alone, for instance, would not provide enough lysine, and a diet which relied heavily on pulses (beans, peas, lentils) would not provide enough of the amino acids which contain sulphur. But a vegetarian diet which included cereals, pulses and nuts would offer the whole range of necessary amino acids.

As for vitamins, vegans and vegetarians tend to consume more vitamin C than the average omnivore, though they may fall short of one or two others. Vitamin A, which our eyes need to function in poor light, is found in animal fats, fish oils and in the pigments of coloured vegetables such as carrots. So a vegan who ate little but rice might find himself stricken with night blindness. Vitamin B_{12} is also missing in vegan diets, and some vegans take vitamin pills containing B_{12} to avoid the kind of anaemia which a deficiency might cause. In fact pernicious anaemia is far from common in people on a vegan diet, and it seems that their lack of B_{12} may be compensated by the relatively large amounts of folic acid they consume in vegetables. Folic acid plays a similar role to B_{12} in the formation of red blood cells. The other vitamin vegetarians may miss is vitamin D, which contributes toward the formation of bones and whose main dietary source is butter, eggs and fish oils. But fortunately this dietary deficiency can be overcome simply by sitting in the sun. Sunlight on the skin converts a body substance, ergosterol, into vitamin D, so deficiency is only likely to affect those who stay indoors or live in a particularly grey climate.

As well as slimness, vegan and vegetarian diets may offer some other healthy advantages. Asians and Africans whose diets are vegetarian suffer hardly at all from the bowel cancers which are relatively common in the Western world, and vegans also have less of the cholesterol and blood fats which are believed to lead to heart disease if they build up excessively in the blood-stream.

Fruitarians, who restrict themselves to fruits, sometimes with the addition of nuts and sprouting seeds like bean sprouts, probably run a greater risk of becoming vitamin-deficient. An ample provision of nuts and seeds would satisfy the body's protein requirements. A tropical fruitarian who was able to get hold of richly pigmented fruits such as mangoes and apricots would be less likely to run low on vitamin A than a northern fruitarian, who would also need to rely on clement weather and sunbathing for supplies of vitamin D.

Young children face more real hazards from this kind of diet, especially if their parents believe that all food should be eaten raw. Young children have more difficulty digesting uncooked proteins than adults, and there have been case reports in medical journals of infants who failed to thrive and grow when their parents kept them to a strict fruitarian diet.

Brown rice has acquired a dubious reputation as the 'wholest of whole foods'. This has largely been due to the popularity of macrobiotic diets, which have been claimed to be a cure for all disease. Macrobiotics draws its inspiration from the old Chinese and Japanese idea that correct living is a matter of balancing the forces of yin and yang. Yin and yang are opposite but inseparable, and stand, among other things, for female and male, water and fire. In the macrobiotic diet, sweet, sour and spicy-tasting foods are generally yin, while bitter or salty foods are yang. Vegetables tend to be yin and meats yang, though there are many gradations between the two poles.

Sick people are encouraged to pursue strict and often extremely limited diets to purify themselves. The boldest claims are made for the most restrictive diet of all, which consists simply of brown rice. Although some devotees may derive spiritual satisfaction from such an austere regime, others have made themselves physically ill. Like honey, which has also been hailed as a cure-all, brown rice is certainly a very nutritious food, but its exclusive use is not to be recommended for anyone who looks forward to a long, vigorous life. Less extreme macrobiotic diets, provided they include a diversity of foods, are probably no better or worse than any other diet which consists of fresh, unprocessed, uncontaminated ingredients.

At their worst, dietary preoccupations have less to do with the pursuit of health than with the devotees' need for a moral or quasi-religious code. Some people are pleased to follow a diet based on ancient Chinese principles which they barely grasp because it makes them feel virtuous. At their best, the diet movements succeed in making people think about what they are eating, the environment it comes from and the environment it is creating inside them.

Of course, the environment has not been completely neglected by modern medicine. Vast population studies have been made of dietary habits and chemical exposures, and they have shown us, among other things, that the risks of heart disease are higher in Western people who eat large amounts of animal fats, and that lung cancer and bronchitis are commoner among people who smoke. Disease can also be caused by a lack of essential nutrients; every enzyme needs its supply of vitamins and trace elements to be able to perform its particular chemical function, and it is well known that a lack of vitamin C is the cause of scurvy, that rickets is caused by a lack of vitamin D and that a lack of vitamin A impairs vision.

The refined carbohydrates white flour and white sugar which make up the bulk of modern diet have been blamed for many chronic diseases, notably bowel cancer and heart disease. I have already described how Dr Francis Hare came to the conclusion that refined carbohydrates were an important factor in obesity and mental disease, but the most famous early critic of our modern, processed foods was Sir Robert McCarrison.

Sir Robert had been a physician working the frontier territory of the British Indian Empire. In the early years of this century he had spent seven years living among the Himalayan Hunza peoples, a race renowned for their longevity and health. In recent years, since Western habits and products have begun to impinge on the lives of these formerly isolated people, their general health has deteriorated and they now seem to be prone to all the 'diseases of civilization'. But fifty years ago McCarrison was very impressed by the Hunzas' physique and vigour, which, he said, were 'unsurpassed by any Indian race'. During his seven years he came across no cases of cancer, peptic ulcer, appendicitis, colitis or gastrointestinal illness, and he wondered how much this might be due to their mountain air and their diet of wholemeal flour, yogurt, cheese and raw vegetables which was washed down with mountain spring water rich in mineral trace elements.

McCarrison was later appointed director of nutrition research in India on the strength of the classic studies he made of dietary factors in disease. When he returned from the Himalayas he set up a series of animal experiments to compare the diets of the Hunzas, the Sikhs of Northern India and the southern Indian population of Madras.

The Sikhs ate a quite similar diet to the Hunzas and were noticeably bigger and healthier than the Madrassis, whose diet contained fewer whole grains and more sugar and more cooked foods. McCarrison experimented on several types of animal — rats, pigeons, guinea pigs, chickens, rabbits and monkeys — and found that those fed on the Hunza and Sikh diets were bigger and healthier in every way than those fed the Madrassi diet. The normal life-span of a laboratory rat is about two years, but McCarrison's rats fed on the Hunza diet lived for five years and remained free of disease. The rats fed the Madrassi diet died sooner and suffered from bad teeth, anaemia, loss of hair, ulcers, crooked spines, skin disease, stomach cancers, rhinits, sinusitis, eye ailments and heart, lung and kidney disorders.

He subsequently compared animals fed on a Sikh diet with animals fed on the diet eaten by poorer, working-class people in Britain, which consisted of white bread, margarine, sweet tea with a little milk, boiled cabbage and potato, and canned meats and jams. Those on the Sikh diet flourished as before, but those on the 'English' diet were stunted and unhealthy, prone to all the metabolic diseases suffered by the Madrassis, and also showed signs of mental disturbance, aggression and an inclination to cannibalism.

Sir Robert McCarrison criticized the Madrassi and the English working-class diets for their reliance on refined grain and sugar. His criticisms have been supported by the more recent investigations of Drs Denis Burkitt and T. L. Cleave, who have shown that bowel cancers, obesity, diabetes, heart disease and several other disorders are rare among peoples whose diets are rich in the natural fibre which is removed when cereals and sugars are refined.

Dietary fibre — which is not the same thing as the stringy fibres found in hemp or string beans — is the material which makes the cell walls in plants. It is indigestible and is not absorbed by the body, so it was once assumed that it had no dietary value and could therefore be discarded. But although fibre is inert, it has important mechanical properties. It traps water, for instance, and by so doing it ensures that the contents of your bowels do not dry up and make you constipated. Free movement in the intestines could reduce the risk of inflammation and the accumulation of toxic substances which may cause cancers and colitis. Fibre also makes food more difficult to eat. This may strike you as a pretty useless property, but the fact is that fibrous foods have to be chewed if we want to extract their flavour and contents. Animals that do not eat refined foods have to chew away at their fruits and nuts, and as they chew their salivary glands produce ample supplies of natural mouthwash, which keeps gums and teeth clean. Animals may wear out their teeth in time, but they do not rot them as we do by eating refined sugars that do not have to be chewed. Dental decay is a relatively new disease which dates from the introduction of refined sugar into the human diet.

I have mentioned the theory that refined carbohydrates are addictive. Dr Ken Heaton, a physician and nutrition researcher at Bristol University, has come up with an alternative theory for obesity. He suggests that the chewability of fibre and its ability to trap liquids makes us feel full more quickly than we would if we were eating refined foods. Writing in *World Medicine,* he explained:

Fibre is unique in that it satiates but does not supply calories. You can test this for yourself by drinking a glass of apple juice and eating two apples. The apples fill you up, the juice leaves you ready to eat. The only difference between the juice and the apples is three grams of fibre. It's astonishing but true that an ordinary eating apple is 98.5 grams of apple juice held together and rendered firm and solid by a mere 1.5 grams of fibre. It's also true that the extra fibre in wholemeal bread provides no energy but people eat fifteen to twenty per cent less whole meal than they do of white bread. Exactly how fibre satiates is not known but it is probably due in part to its hardening effect on food texture. When apples are made into a purée, they are less satisfying than the whole fruit.

In other words, fibre discourages us from eating more than we need. Dr Heaton has tested this idea by getting one group of volunteers to eat an unrefined carbohydrate diet consisting of whole wheat bread, plentiful fruit and vegetables with no refined sugar, and another group to follow a diet in which the carbohydrate was all refined — white bread, cakes made of white flour and plenty of sugar and sugary foods. The volunteers were told to eat as much as they wanted, but not to overeat. After seven weeks all the volunteers on the refined diet had put on weight while all the volunteers on the unrefined diet lost weight. An analysis of their daily intake of calories revealed that the volunteers on the refined flour and sugar diet were consuming 484 calories (the equivalent of an average lunch) more than the other group.

Cooking, it seems, may also drastically reduce the nutritional value of foods. I have already mentioned in Chapter 3 how a researcher found that frozen processed chicken and vegetable pies sold in supermarkets had lost all their orginal vitamin C by the time they reached the consumer's plate. The American medical researcher Francis Pottenger discovered something even more alarming when he compared cats which had been fed raw food with cats which had been fed cooked food. The cats which were given raw meat and unpasteurized milk grew, bred and lived their lives with every sign of good health. Mother cats gave birth to an average of five kittens a time which they suckled normally. All the animals had a normal or better than average resistance to infections and parasites.

The other cats, who were fed cooked meats and pasteurized or boiled milk, did not do so well. As Pottenger reported:

> Abortion in these cats was common, running at about 25 per cent in the first generation to about 70 per cent in the second generation. Deliveries were in general difficult; many cats died in labour. Mortality rates of the kittens were high, freqently due to the failure of the mother to lactate. The kittens were often too frail to nurse. At times the mother would steadily decline in health following the birth of the kittens, dying from some obscure tissue exhaustion about three months after delivery. Others experienced increasing difficulty with subsequent pregnancies. Some failed to become pregnant, although for all breeding purposes we used a normal, raw meat-fed male of proven fecundity, thus eliminating the possibility of male sterility.
>
> Cats fed cooked meat were irritable. The females were dangerous to handle, occasionally viciously biting the handler. The males were more docile, often to the point of being unaggressive. Sex interest was slack or perverted. Vermin and intestinal parasites abounded. Skin lesions and allergies were frequent, being progressively worse from one generation to the next. Pneumonia and empyema [lung abscesses] were among the principal causes of natural death among the adult cats. Diarrhoea followed by pneumonia took a heavy toll of the kittens; osteomyelitis [abscesses in the bone marrow] was also both common and often fatal. Cardiac lesions were frequent. Myopia [short sight], thyroid disease, nephritis [kidney disease], hepatitis [liver disease], orchitis [inflamed testicles], oophoritis [inflamed ovaries], paralysis, meningitis, cystitis, arthritis and many others degenerative lesions familiar in human medicine were observed.

A pretty horrific inventory, and one which may make the devoted pet lover think twice before giving kitty a hot supper. But cats is cats and people is people. We are more used to cooked food than kitties are, so what is the evidence that cooking is harmful for us?

Although cooking does destroy vitamins and other nutrients it is sometimes essential. Infants find it hard to digest protein and do better on lightly cooked food. Kidney beans and black beans contain haemagglutinin, a class of protein which poisons the blood, but is destroyed by cooking.

Some cooking methods, however, do appear to increase the amount of substances in food which can cause cancer. When meat is grilled or smoked some of the proteins are changed into substances called polycyclic aromatic hydrocarbons, which despite their appealing name are known to be carcinogenic. Icelanders who live in remote parts where vegetables are unavailable eat a diet which consists largely of smoked fish and seabirds. These people are particularly prone to stomach cancers, and this has been attributed to the large quantities of polycyclic aromatic hydrocarbons they ingest. And a research team at Washington University, Missouri, discovered in 1978 that 'well done' hamburgers contained much larger amounts of a mutagen (a potentially carcinogenic substance) than 'rare' hamburgers. This substance could also be created by boiling beef stock down to the paste from which bouillon cubes are made. The original beef barely contained any of this substance, but after it had been boiled for ten hours the mutagen content was sixty times higher.

Of course, it is easy to get overly concerned about poisons in food. Nearly all fresh, natural foods contain trace quantities of toxic substances which have nothing to do with contamination from pesticides or fertilizers. Seafood contains up to 150 parts per million of arsenic, but arsenic poisoning in seafood enthusiasts is apparently unknown.

Even the much maligned food additives may not be all bad. Dr Lee Wattenburg, professor of pathology at the Unversity of Minnesota, recently discovered from animal tests that BHA (butylated hydroxyanisole — an antioxidant which is added to butter and other foods to prevent their fats from going rancid) can actually counteract the carcinogenic effect of nitrosamines and polycyclic hydrocarbons. A related chemical, BHT (butylated hydroxytoluene, which is added to 'instant' potato) also has this effect, but only if it is taken *before* the animal is exposed to the carcinogen. If the animal ingests BHT *after* being exposed to the carcinogen, the additive actually increases the cancer risk.

It would take a million years to work out the possible risks and/or benefits caused by the interaction of natural and artificial dietary chemicals. And whether we like it or not, we are all guinea pigs in this vast experiment. The main aim of this book, however, is to point out that food and chemical allergy is something which affects *individuals* rather than whole populations. A poor diet or exposure to a chemical may increase the chances of disease, but it does not guarantee it. Not every smoker gets lung cancer, nor does every Icelander who eats smoked seagull get stomach cancer. A very few people are allergic to BHT and their lips and tongue will swell when they as much as taste a morsel of instant mashed potato containing BHT. But they have probably been no more exposed to BHT than other members of their family who do not appear to react at all badly to the stuff. Lots of salt in the diet increases the likelihood that you will get high blood-pressure; but Sir George Pickering, a British physician who refused to accept this theory, proved that likelihood was not certainty: at every available opportunity he would publicly demonstrate his disbelief by smothering his food in salt and relishing every mouthful. He did not get high blood-pressure.

Food and chemical allergies are an individual's response to the environment, and they depend on genetic background, mother's diet, how often you are exposed to the allergen, your general health and your unique biochemistry. Many doctors have tried to lay down rules saying what allergy is and what it is not. But interesting though the theories may be, they never seem to provide a complete answer.

Immunological Classification of Allergies

In 1968 two British immunologists, Drs Gell and Coombs, classified allergic reactions into four types.

Type One reactions are caused by antigens descending on mast cells which have been coated with the antibody IgE. When this happens, the interaction between the antibody and the antigen makes the mast cell release inflammatory substances, notably histamine. The symptoms of such a reaction come on quickly, reaching a peak after fifteen to twenty minutes and lasting for about two hours. In the skin the symptoms take the form of itching, redness and wealing. In the air passages and the digestive tract the inflammatory substances released by the mast cells prompt the mucous membranes to produce large quantities of mucus. The symptoms generally though not always manifest themselves in the area where cells have been coated with IgE. So someone who has antibody to pollen attached to mast cells in the tissues of his nose will get rhinitis when exposed to pollen, while someone whose digestive tract has been sensitized to a food allergen is likely to get diarrhoea when he eats that food.

Type Two reactions are the result of an antigen attaching itself to a tissue cell penetrating into the blood-stream, where it latches on to a red blood cell (the kind of cell which transports oxygen). With this foreign passenger riding on its back the cell attracts antibodies which destroy it. If the antigen is attached to red blood cells the patient can eventually become anaemic because the red cells are being destroyed faster than they can be created. Sometimes the antigen attaches itself to platelets, the 'sticky' cells which adhere to each other and plug gaps in the walls of blood vessels when they are damaged. If large numbers of platelets are knocked out by antibodies, the body's self-healing mechanism is upset and the patient may bruise very easily.

A number of drugs can cause Type Two reactions, including methyl-dopa, a medicine commonly prescribed for treating high blood-pressure.

Type Three   reactions are the result of the immune system going off at half cock. Antibodies descend upon allergens, but do not succeed in destroying them completely. So the allergen and antibody are left locked in what is called an 'immune complex'. As well as antibodies there are a number of cells (macrophages) and proteins (complement) which also drift around the system clearing up unwanted micro-organisms and other nasty messes such as immune complexes. They move in to destroy the immune complex, but in doing so they produce destructive enzymes which burn away the complex and the tissue surrounding it.

Agricultural workers and other country people who are exposed to damp hay sometimes develop a complaint called 'farmer's lung'. This is an allergic reaction to a spore from a fungus which grows in warm, damp hay and it leads to chronic inflammation of the lungs. This disease has been described as the consequence of a Type Three allergic reaction. Stomach ulcers have also been blamed on milk and other foods causing a Type Three reaction. The thinking behind this is that if the stomach lining of a patient who drinks a lot of milk has somehow become sensitized to an antigen in milk, regular indigestion of milk will cause a build-up of immune complexes on the sensitized area, which will eventually become inflamed.

I mentioned that in Type One allergic reactions, the class of antibody involved was called IgE. In Type Two and Type Three the antibodies involved are IgG and IgM. The difference between these antibodies is in their chemical structure, which in turn determines what kind of tissue they latch on to. Broadly speaking, though, their functions are similar. There is another class of antibody, IgA, which is found largely in the walls of the gut, where it is believed to act as a kind of filter, intercepting large molecules of anitgen before they can break through the gastrointestinal lining into the blood-stream. It seems that it is only when antigens somehow push through this defensive line of IgA that they set the allergic process in action by drawing the attention of the other kinds of antibody. The reason why babies sometimes develop an allergy to cow's milk is that their system has not had time to produce this kind of antibody. Protein molecules from the foreign milk are therefore able to get into the blood-stream, where they eventually cause IgE antibodies to be produced.

If they are produced in sufficiently large quantities, they attach themselves to mast cells in the gut, so that when the allergen comes by again it sparks off a Type One reaction, giving the baby diarrhoea and colic.

Type Four reactions are the result of an antibody becoming attached to white cells (lymphocytes) which lodge in tissues rather than the blood-stream. When exposed to an allergen, the sensitized lymphocytes produce substances called lymphokines which set off local inflammation. The commonest kind of Type Four reaction is *contact dermatitis*, the itchy skin rash some people get when they come into contact with a substance to which they have somehow become sensitized. All kinds of substances can cause contact dermatitis: some people get it from the rubber in the elastic of their underclothes, others suffer when they handle certain metals, and sometimes cosmetics are to blame. Housewives have developed contact dermatitis from washing powders. Contact dermatitis is a delayed reaction which may take a day or two to reveal itself. It is therefore quite distinct from *atopic dermatitis*, which occurs very soon after exposure to the allergen and is mediated by IgE. Contact dermatitis also tends to be confined to the site of contact with the allergen, whereas atopic dermatitis can appear almost anywhere on the body. Food allergy is one cause of atopic dermatitis. There are several kinds of dermatitis, and they are sometimes lumped together under the general title of `eczema' even though they are different forms of allergic reaction.

The great puzzle about allergies is why some people are adversely affected by a substance which is quite harmless to the majority of us. Although allergies do tend to run in families, the pattern of inheritance is unclear. However, immunologists have recently suggested that people with Type One allergies may have an abnormality in their white cells. Antibody is produced by a kind of white cell called the B-lymphocyte. Now, there is another kind of lymphocyte, the T-lymphocyte, which cannot produce antibody but is able to attack foreign antigens directly. To destroy the antigen the T-lymphocyte releases substances called lymphokines, and it seems that lymphokines can influence the way the B-lymphocyte reacts to the antigen. Thus, if the T-lymphocytes encounter an antigen they regard as a threat to the body, the lymphokines they release will encourage the B-lymphocytes to produce antibody. If, however, the T-lymphocytes encounter an antigen which does not apper to present a threat, they release substances which prevent the B-lymphocytes from producing antibody. Depending on whether they switch on B-lymphocytes to produce antibody or prevent them from so doing, T-lymphocytes have been described as 'helper' and 'suppressor' cells.

A recent theory is that allergic people lack an effective 'suppressor' cell mechanism, which means that there is nothing to stop the B-lymphocytes from producing large amounts when faced by a harmless antigen.

Whether this theory will stand up in the light of future research remains to be seen. It is still, of course, just an explanation of one aspect of a complex, poorly understood and highly controversial subject.

Appendix II:

A Review of Methods for Diagnosing and Treating Food Allergy

1. Individual feeding test

If you suspect that a particular food is making you feel unwell, give it up for at least five days, and then feed yourself generously with it. If your symptoms disappear when you avoid the food and reappear when you eat it again (remember the effects may be delayed for as long as four days), you have probably identified the culprit. Do not eat it again for a few months, then try it again: some food allergies can be eradicated if you avoid the food for long enough. But don't forget what happened to Dr Rinkel! (see pages 41-2). Reactions to re-exposure can be acute.

2. Elimination diet

Refer back to page 36 for a detailed explanation of the elimination diets used by various doctors. You can be allergic to any food or chemical, it seems, but the main foods you should exclude from your diet are eggs; cereals (foods made from wheat, corn, barley, oats, rice, millet, especially any cereal which you eat regularly); beer and whisky; milk and dairy products (e.g., cheese, yogurt, butter); coffee and tea; *all* canned, frozen, processed and preserved foods, including chocolate and fish. Meats seem to be less allergenic than these foods, but it would be wise to confine yourself to one kind of meat at a time. Once you find a basic diet which relieves your symptoms, stick to it until the symptoms clear then add individual foods one by one.

3. Pulse test

You can use the pulse tests after eating a food or after taking an under-the-tongue drop of mashed food or food extract. You feel your pulse by putting your index and second fingers on the thickest artery on the front of your wrist, about an inch down from where your hand joins your arm. Take your pulse before feeding (it will probably be steady at around seventy beats a minute) and take it again five, ten and thirty minutes after feeding. Again, the reaction can be delayed, so a rapid acceleration or deceleration may not occur for an hour or two after eating. A sublingual test will generally produce much quicker effects. A change in pulse is usually the sign of more severe reactions to come. These can be prevented by taking a spoonful of bicarbonate of soda in a large mug of warm water if you have eaten the food, or by a 1:100 or 1:1,000 dilution of extract if you have done a sublingual test.

4. Sublingual and intradermal 'switch-on/switch off'

An ambitious self-diagnostician might try to make his own food extracts for under-the-tongue tests, but this is probably best left to experienced medical ecologists who know what they are doing. Intradermal injections are certainly just for the expert. Interpreting the significance of a reaction from the size and shape of the weal is an art which requires practice. Switch-offs are performed by injecting 1:25, 1:125, 1:625 or smaller dilution of the extract.

5. Drugs

Drugs such as antihistamine or sodium cromoglycate are taken before exposure to an allergen to 'block' the reaction. They are only available on prescription.

Appendix III:

Food Families

If you are allergic to a food, you may also be allergic to other foods in the same biological family, This is a list of the more common related foods.

1. wheat, corn, sweetcorn, barley, oats, rye, millet, sugar cane
2. coconut, sago, dates
3. asparagus, onions, chives, garlic, yucca
4. rhubarb, buckwheat
5. cinnamon, avocados
6. cabbage, cauliflower, kale, Brussels sprouts, mustard, turnips
7. blackberries, strawberries, raspberries, loganberries
8. apples, plums (and prunes), pears, cherries, apricots, almonds
9. liquorice, lentils, soya beans, peanuts, broad beans, haricot beans, kidney beans, peas
10. lemons, limes, oranges, grapefruit, mandarins, ugli fruits
11. cashews, pistachios, mangoes
12. carrots, celery, parsnips, fennel, dill, aniseed, caraway seeds, angelica
13. potatoes, tobacco, aubergines, tomatoes, green peppers
14. peppermint, spearmint, basil, lavender, rosemary, majoram, sage, savory, thyme
15. cucumbers, watermelons
16. lettuce, endives, chicory, artichokes (common and Jerusalem), sunflower, dandelion, camomile, safflower
17. walnuts, pecan nuts, hickory nuts
18. hazelnuts, filberts, wintergreens
19. oysters, clams, scallops, mussels
20. shrimp, lobsters, crabs, crayfish

Appendix IV:

Hidden Foods

1. *Wheat* and/or *corn* flour is added to a vast array of foods. Meat pies, sausages, mustard powder, garlic salt, soup, instant coffee, mayonnaise may all contain flour as a makeweight. The only answer is to avoid these foods when you are on an exclusion diet.
2. *Milk and eggs* are equally common.
3. *Fish proteins* are a common ingredient of glues — so beware of postage stamps and envelopes which need licking. The tongue is an extremely sensitive allergen receptor.
4. *Soya beans* go into the making of soy sauce, margarines, Worcestershire sauce, monosodium glutamate, Chinese food, toffees and caramels, cooking oils — and are now widely used as meat substitutes or extenders. Industry uses soya products for making — among other things — animal food, candles, fertilizers, glues, pesticides, resins and varnishes. They might present a problem to an allergic person working in a factory which manufactures such products.
5. *Salicylates:* Aspirin sensitivity usually reveals itself as a wheeze when aspirin is taken to relieve pain or fever, though it can also cause rashes and other allergic symptoms. Breathing problems would probably first be noticed an hour or two after taking the aspirin.

People who are allergic to aspirin are usually just sensitive to the 'acetyl' part of acetylsalcylic acid though some are sensitive to all salicylates. Salicylates often crop up in food flavourings, chewing gum, soft and fizzy drinks, toothpaste, mouthwash, suntan lotions, lozenges, ice-cream and jams and jellies. This may not be mentioned on the label, so the best advice if you are not sure is to avoid the product.

The commonest natural sources of salicylates are almonds, apples, apricots, blackberries, cherries, cucumbers and dill pickles, currants, gooseberries, grapes (and raisins), nectarines, oranges, peaches, plums (and prunes), raspberries, strawberries and tomatoes.

The willow tree was the original source of pain-killing medicines made from salicylates, and the leaves, bark, fruits, flowers and stems of willow and the following plants contain salicylates: acacia, aspen, birch, poplar, hyacinth, marigold, camelia, tulip, violet, teaberry, calcanthus, spiraea and milkwort.

Salicylates are very common in medicines you can buy over the counter from a pharmacist.

Appendix V:

Additives

I said in Chapter 3 that there were about three thousand synthetic and natural chemicals which are now used for flavouring, preserving, colouring, stabilizing and performing other actions on foods. This is no place for a list of all those substances or for a detailed description of what each does. However, you might find it useful to know what the commonest additives are, what they do, and where you can expert to find them. Anyone who wants a little more background information could turn to a book called *Why Additives?* which was edited by the British Nutrition Foundation and published by Forbes Publications (1977). This book is generally 'pro' additives and takes pains to stress that we are not all at risk from their presence. A much more 'anti' additives book is the American publication *Food Additives and Your Health*, by Beatrice Trum Hunter, published by Keats Publishing, New Canaan, Connecticut, which goes into detail about the known hazards of the principal additives. Both these books are inexpensive paperbacks.

A book which lists additives according to the new EEC 'E' numbers is especially useful now that these numbers are used on food labels. It is called *E for Additives* by M. Hanssen, published by Thorsons Publishing Group.

Acids
Acids are added to foods mainly to give them a sharp taste. The commonest are citric acid, malic acid, tartaric acid, acetic acid and lactic acid. All these also occur naturally in various fruits and vegetables, or, in the case of lactic acid, in sour milk and yogurt. In processed foods they are often added to jams, sweets and soft drinks.

Some more potent acids such as phosphoric acid and hydrochloric acid are also permitted additives.

Alkalis and Bases
These are added to neutralize excess or unwanted acids. They are sometimes added to wines, for instance, to stop them from becoming too sharp-tasting. Chalk and bicarbonate of soda are widely used to counteract acidity. Chalk is in fact a *compulsory* additive to plain white flour in Britain. It was originally introduced to improve the population's calcium intake, though the justification for its continued addition is dubious, as calcium shortage is hardly a problem in modern diets. *Antioxidants* are added to oils and fats to stop them from going rancid when exposed to the oxygen in the air. As many cooking processes involve the use of fats and oils, antioxidants find their way into most processed foods, as well as into commercial brands of butter, margarine, lard and cooking oil. The main antioxidants are butylated hydroxytoluene (BHT), butylated hydroxyanisole (BHA) and substances called gallates. BHT is known to cause rashes and other allergic reactions in a small number of people. Another antioxidant, ethoxyquin, causes severe eczema in people who handled it, though not apparently in those who ate it. It is no longer permitted in Britain and the European Economic Community.

Bleaches
Benzoyl peroxide is added to flour to whiten it.

Buffers
A buffer is an additive which modifies the acidity or alkalinity of foods or drinks. See under *Acids* and *Alkalis and Bases*.

Colours and Dyes
These are probably the riskiest group for allergy-prone people and have little value except to deceive the eye and improve the appearance of foods. Tartrazine (a yellow dye) and the dye 'sunset yellow' can cause a variety of allergic reactions including skin rashes and asthma. Several dyes which were once regarded as safe have recently been banned in Britain, the United States and the EEC,

though more because of possible cancer risks than due to their allergenic properties.

Many pills and medicines are also coloured. A few allergic patients have actually got worse after being prescribed tablets containing red or yellow dye, and some patients taking antibiotics have developed rashes which were caused by a sensitivity to tartrazine rather than to the antibiotic itself.

Preservatives

Preservatives are added to foods to prevent or delay spoilage, the growth of moulds or the growth of dangerous bacteria. Without them food would undoubtedly be more expensive, because large amounts would go 'bad' before being bought and consumed. Sadly, however, some preservatives do cause allergic reactions and others have been suspected as possible causes of cancer.

The commonest preservatives are the sodium nitrates and nitrates, benzoic acid and the benzoates, sulphur dioxide and propionic acid. The nitrates (nitrates are broken down into nitrites by bacteria) are primarily added to meats, especially those which are canned or pressed. They are also used as fertilizers, and find their way into the water supply when they are washed off the fields by rain. Their great virtue is that they check the growth of the organism which causes botulism, an extremely dangerous disease. However, they have also been suspected as being a cancer risk, because in the body nitrites are changed into nitrosamines, which are potent carcinogens. How much of a risk is presented by the small quantities in foods is not yet known.

Emulsifiers and Stabilizers

Emulsifiers allow oily and watery substances to be mixed together without separating. The best example of an emulsifier is the egg yolk we use in mayonnaise to keep the oil and vinegar together. (The actual ingredient in egg yolk responsible for this is lecithin.) After a while emulsions will separate, so stabilizers are added to delay this occurrence.

Emulsifiers are able to hold oil and water together because they have opposing characteristics within the same molecule. One 'end' of the molecule is attracted to oil, but hates water, while the other 'end' hates oil, but loves water. The emulsifier therefore forms a link between the oil and water, with its head attached to the one and its tail attached to the other.

Natural, and, more commonly, synthetic emulsifiers and stabilizers are added to cake, bread and batter mixes, to ice-cream and to confections like chocolate, where they prevent the cocoa butter separating from the chocolate. (This separation makes chocolate develop a whitish bloom when it is exposed to temperature changes.)

Flavourings

Natural and synthetic flavouring agents account for around two thousand of the additives which go into food today. Natural flavours are derived directly from plants, herbs and fruits, and they are usually either essential oils or resins. Essential oils are generally extracted by distillation, while resins are extracted with the help of solvents.

Many flavourings are derived from natural, organic sources, though not from the fruit or spice we associate with that flavour. For instance, the distinctive taste of vanilla lies in the substance vanillin, which is found not only in vanilla pods but also in some wood fibres. Vanillin can be extracted from pulped wood much more cheaply than it can be obtained from vanilla pods. So the vanilla essence sold in bottles in the supermarket is almost always a by-product of the paper industry. Or it could be entirely synthetic. Scientists might argue that this vanillin is extremely pure, though anyone who has compared the taste of vanilla pods with that of vanilla essence will know that the pod's flavour is infinitely more subtle and delightful. Chemical purity is not necessarily a virtue!

The distinctive flavour of lemon comes from citral, which can also be derived, at low cost, from lemongrass. This plant is therefore a much commoner source of lemon flavouring than the fruit.

Solvents

As most flavourings are highly concentrated they are often added to a solvent to ensure that they can be spread uniformly through the food to which they are being added. Water dissolves many salts, alcohol dissolves most resins and ether dissolves fats. In a lot of packaged foods, however, liquid flavourings are mixed with salt, edible gum or starch before being added to the food.

Sulphur dioxide, hydrobenzoic acid and the benzoates are added to beer, soft and fizzy drinks, wine, sausages, dried fruit and vegetables and jams, among other things. Sulphur dioxide is a potent allergen and tiny quantities can produce strong asthmatic and/or skin reactions in sensitive people. Hydrobenzoic acid can have a similar effect on a few of us.

Propionic acid is added mainly to bread and cakes to stop them from going mouldy.

Air Excluders

Nitrogen, hydrogen or carbon dioxide are sometimes pumped into food packages to prevent the food inside coming into contact with the air and thus becoming rancid or mouldy. Foods can also be 'quick frozen' by liquid nitrogen.

Anti-stick Substances

Beeswax is used as a polish on pills and some foods. Magnesium carbonate is added to table salt to prevent it from forming into lumps.

Phosphates

Phosphates usually lie behind the term 'emulsifying salts' found on some food labels. In this context they are added to milk during the production of processed cheese to stop the milk fats from separating from the watery liquid. Similarly they have an effect on meat proteins which discourages fat and meat juices running out during cooking.

Acid calcium phosphate (ACP) is an ingredient of baking powder. Its acid action is delayed, which allows the powder to have a sustained effect on the dough or batter as it is cooked.

Humectants

Humectants keep foods moist and prevent their becoming undesirably hard or brittle. Glycerine is often added to cake icing for this purpose. Sorbitol, which is chemically similar to the sugars, is another commonly used humectant.

Sequestrants

Also known as chelating agents or metal scavengers, sequestrants are added to foods to remove traces of metals like copper and iron, whose presence, even in tiny amounts, can accelerate rancidity and spoilage. The commonest, calcium disodium EDTA, is added to a wide variety of foods. It is also used to treat people suffering from lead poisoning. The principal hazard of sequestrants is that they have the potential to upset the body's natural chemical balance by removing vital trace elements.

This is only a bare outline of food additives. Although perhaps less than one person in a thousand reacts very strongly to such chemicals, chemical sensitivity is a subject which has only just begun to be explored by scientists. I commented on its complexity in Chapter 3.

Regulations about labelling foods are also very complicated and vary from country to country. Anyone who does have a sensitivity to, say, hydrobenzoic acid, is not likely to be helped by a food label which states that 'permitted preservatives' have been added but does not specify which ones. At present it seems that the only sure way of identifying a chemical allergy is to eat foods which are as uncontaminated as possible. If these do not make you sick, then try commercial or processed varieties which have been treated with additives to see if you get a reaction.

REFERENCES AND FURTHER READING

Several case histories and reports of scientific and clinical studies have been taken from published books and papers. These include:

Bray, G., *Recent Advances in Allergy* (London: Churchill, 1934).

Breneman, J. C., *Basics of Food Allergy* (Springfield, Ill.: Thomas, 1978).

Coca, A., *The Pulse Test* (New York: Arco, 1956).

Dickey, L. D., ed. *Clinical Ecology* (Springfield, Ill.: Thomas, 1976).

Hall, R. H., *Food for Nought* (New York: Harper and Row, 1974).

Hare, F., *The Food Factor in Disease* (London: Longmans, 1906).

Mackarness, R., *Not All in the Mind* (London: Pan, 1976).

Randolph, T. G., *Human Ecology and Susceptibility to the Chemical Environment* (Springfield, Ill.: Thomas, 1962).

Rapp, Doris, and Frankland, A. W., *Allergies: Questions and Answers* (London: William Heineman Medical Bks., 1976).

Journals

Lancet. Several papers and letters in 1978 and 1979 on food allergy, notably in issues of:
11 February 1978 (Buisseret); 25 February 1978 (Finn, Cohen); 18 March 1978 (Hemmings); 8 April 1978 (Dickerson et al.); 29 April 1978 (Buisseret); 24 June 1978 (Ellis, Linaker); 26 August 1978 (Jakobsson, Lindberg); 9 September 1978 (Grant); 7 October 1978 (Jackson, Golden); 11 October 1978 (Logan, Ferguson, Offord); 3 February 1979 (leading article); 5 May 1979 (Grant); 5 December 1979 (Dohan).

Practitioner, Symposium on Allergy, April 1978.

Journal of Human Nutrition, Symposium on Nutrition, May 1979; Symposium issue on 'Allergy and the gut', June 1976.

Conferences

13th Annual Meeting of the Society for Clinical Ecology, November 1978. (Abstracts obtained from L. D. Dickey, M.D., 109 West Olive, Fort Collins, Colorado.)

Clinical Ecology Seminar sponsored by Society for Clinical Ecology at Royal College of Physicians, London, May 1979.

Index

aches and pains, 96-7
acids, 182-3
ACTH (adrenocorticotropic
  hormone), 44
acupuncture, 141
addiction, 98
addiction, food, 147-51: see also
  compulsive eating; obesity
additives, 55-71, 98, 130-31,
  182-7
adrenalin, 31, 81, 112
adrenocorticotropic hormone,
  see ACTH
Adresen, A.F.R., 37
aerosols, 102
aflatoxins, 101
air excluders, 186
airborne allergens, 100-102
albumin, 65
alcohol, 63, 67-8, 134
alcoholism, 14, 146-54
alkalis, 183
allergens, 30-31, 70, 82, 98; and
  passim
allergic toxaemia, 37
allergy theory: history, 13-25
allergy, masked, 97-8
almonds, 100, 129
aluminium, 103, 127
Amoco Food Company, 65
anaemia, 83
anaphylaxis, 81-2
anger, 101
angina, 33, 96, 151
anti-stick substances, 186
antibiotics, 83, 100-101
antibodies, 13-14, 29-30, 70,
  73-4
antidepressants, 64
antigens, 13-14, 29, 82
antihistamines, 19, 57, 111-12
anxiety, 101
appetite-suppressant drugs,
  146-7
apples, 100, 129, 159
apricots, 100
arachidonic acid, 109
Archives of Internal Medicine, 34
arsenic, 128
arteries, hardening of, 96
arthritis, 14-16, 33, 83, 96, 151,
  155-61: see also rheumatoid
  arthritis
aspirin, 100, 108, 110-11, 129
asthma, 14, 27, 30, 33, 35, 37,
  56-7, 71, 89, 96, 101, 113,
  128-9, 131, 151
atmospheric pollution, 10, 147
aubergines, 100

Austria, 29
autoimmunity, 83, 155-6

B-lymphocytes, 29; see also
  blood cells
bacteria, 29
Baker, P.G., 124
bananas, 110, 119
barbiturates, 63
barley, 122
beans, 100
beans, black, 171
beans, broad, 97, 133
beans, butter, 159
beans, kidney, 171
bed-wetting, 14, 96, 119-21
beef, 10, 48, 100, 135, 159
beer, 110
Bencard, 90-91
berries, 89, 100
beta-glucuronidase, 92
betalactoglobulin, 115
BHA (butylated
  hydroxyanisole), 171
BHT (butylated
  hydroxytoluene), 171-2
Biorex, 91
Blackley, Dr Charles, 26-7
bleaches, 183
blood cells, 29
blood serum, 27-8
blood-pressure, high, 33, 96,
  151
Board of Allergy and
  Immunology, 28
Bray, George, 120
bread, 59-60; see also individual
  cereals
breast-feeding, 73-4; see also
  milk
Breneman, J.C., 149; Basics of
  Food Allergy, 99, 120-21,
  137, 148
Brisbane, 33
Britain, Great, 28, 37-8, 90,
  128; see also individual
  towns and cities
British Medical Journal, 62, 124,
  144, 147
British Medicine (journal), 25
British National Formulary, the,
  147
bronchitis, 33, 96, 151
Brostoff, Jonathan, 80
Bruff, Jane, 16-18, 20-21
Bryce-Smith, Derek, 127
buffers, 183
Buisseret, P.D., 109, 111
Burkitt, Denis, 168

Burton, Robert, The Anatomy of
  Melancholy, 132
Buscaino, V.M., and G.A., 142
butter, 60

Cade, Dr, 143
cadmium, 128
calcium deficiency, 120
Cambridge, Massachusetts, 67
can linings, 102
cancer, 14, 96, 171
carbohydrates, 51, 151
Cardiothoracic Institute,
  London, 69
Carroll, F. Murray, 159-60
case histories, 15-23
Casper, Billy, 9-11
Casper, Mrs Billy, 9-11
catarrh, 37
catastrophic anaphylaxis, 31
catatonia, 101
cereal, 54; see also grains;
  individual cereals
Charing Cross Hospital,
  London, 133
cheese, 89, 97, 133-4, 136
chemical allergies, 11-12, 69-71,
  93-4, 102-7, 128-31, 161
chemical contamination,
  47-50, 68
chewing gum, 100
Chicago, 105
chicken pox, 29
chicken, 10-11, 100
Chinese Restaurant syndrome,
  57-8
chlorine, 106
chocolate, 97, 133-6, 159
Chvostek reflex, the, 120-21
cigarette smoking, 133-4
Clark, Sue, 22-3
Cleave, T.L., 168
Coca, Dr Arthur, 38-40, 42, 63;
  Familial Non-Reaginic Food
  Allergy, 39; The Pulse Test, 40
Coca-Cola, 111; see also cola
  drinks
coeliac disease, 71-3, 122-5,
  131, 140, 142
Coeliac Society, the, 124
coffee, 100, 135, 159
cola drinks, 159
colic, 14, 96
colitis, ulcerative, 37, 96
College of Allergists (US), 77
colouring, 62-4, 183-4
Committee on the Safety of
  Medicines (British), 56
concentration, lack of, 96

conjunctivitis, 96
Connor, Mary, 19-20
convulsions, 96
Coombs, Dr, 173
corn, 65, 67-8, 98, 100, 110,
  135, 139-40, 159
corticosteroid hormones, 52
cosmetics, 100
Crook, William, Can Your Child
  Read? 127
cyclamate sweeteners, 58
cyclohexane, 92-3
cystitis, 122
Czechoslovakia, 89

Dallas, 105
danders, animal, 100
degenerative diseases, 33, 151
Delaney clause, the, 58
Department of Agriculture
  (US), 61, 63, 66
Department of Health (UK),
  146-7
depression, 14, 96, 101, 132
desensitization, 75-107
diagnosis, 75-107, 177-8
dialysis, 142-3
diarrhoea, 96, 109-10
Dicke, W.K., 123
Dickerson, J.W.T., 136
Dickey, Larry, 102-3
diet, 84-9, 162-72: see also
  elimination diets; exclusion
  diets
dietary fibre, 168-9
diethylstilboestrol hormone, 64
diphtheria, 29
disinfectants, 102
disodium cromoglycate, 112
Dohan, F. Curtis, 139-40
Donaldson, Blake, 150
dopamine, 138
drugs, 64, 102, 108-13, 178; see
  also medicines
Duke, Dr William, 34, 120
Durrant, Barry, 144
dust, 30
dust mites, 100
dyes, 64, 128-9, 183-4
dyslexia, 71-3

ears, ringing in, 96
eating, compulsive, 146; see also
  obesity
ecological medicine, 28, 32-54
ecologists, clinical, 98, 105, 151
eczema, 14, 33, 35, 37, 71, 89,
  96-7, 151
eggs, 31-2, 34-5, 41-2, 54, 65,

70, 84, 89, 97-8, 100, 110,
  118, 136
electrical stimulation, 141
elimination diet, 36, 99-100,
  177; see also exclusion diets
emulsifiers, 184-5
endorphins, 138-43, 148
England, see Britain, Great
Entero-Vioform, 83-4, 88
enzymes, 71, 91, 97, 109; see
  also individual types
epilepsy, 33, 71, 149
epileptic fits, 97; see also fits
epinephrine, 81
ergot, 101
ergotamine, 134
ethanol, 105
exclusion diets, 81, 110, 134-7;
  see also elimination diets
exhaust fumes, 102
exorphins, 142, 148-9

fabrics, plastic, 103
fainting, 96
fat, animal, 118
Feingold, Ben, 127, 129-31
fertilizers, 59
fibre, see dietary fibre
Finn, Ronald, 20-23, 132-3,
  135, 154
fish, 31-2, 81-2, 84, 89, 118
fits, 96
flame retardants, 103
flavourings, 128-9, 185
flour, 65
fluorine, 106
Fomon, Dr S.J., Infant Nutrition,
  118
Food Additives and
  Contaminants Committee
  (Britain), 63
food allergies, 10, 27, 29-31,
  33-54, 71-4, and passim; see
  also specific foods
Food and Drug Administration
  (US), 63
food extract, 75-6, 79
food families, 179
food technology, 66
Frankland, A.W. see Rapp.
  Doris, and A.W. Frankland
Frankland, Bill, 30, 57, 81-2, 88
Freed, David, 144
Freedman, Bernard, 57
Freeman, J., 27, 82
Freon, 12, 63
fruit, 89, 129
fruit, citrus, 100, 134
fruitarians, 165

gallstones, 96
gas, 102
gastrointestinal disturbances,
  33
Gee, Samuel, 122-3
Gell, Dr, 173
General Medical Council
  (British), 90
Germany, 29
Gerrard, John, 115, 121
globulin, 65
gluten, 122-5
Golden, Dr Michael, 115-17
gout, 33, 151, 155
grains, refined, 118
Grant, Ellen, 133-5
Guy's Hospital, London, 109

haemagglutinin, 171
Hall, Ross Hume, Food for
  Nought, 66
Hannington, Edda, 133
haptens, 71
Hare, Francis, 51, 166; The Food

Factor in Disease, 32-3, 151;
  On Alcoholism, 151
hay fever, 14, 26-7, 30, 79-80,
  83, 112
headaches, 101
heart disease, 96
Heaton, Ken, 168-9
Hemmings, W.A., 144, 150
hepatitis, 29, 137
herbicides, 59
heredity, and allergies, 115
herrings, pickled, 97
hidden foods, 180-81
Hippocrates, 13
histamine, 13, 111
hives, 38, 96
Hockett, Dr, 67
hormones, 44, 52, 60, 64, 112
Hospital for Sick Children,
  London, 135-6
Hughes, John, 141
humectants, 186
hunger, 134
Hunzas, 167
hyaluronidase, 91-2
hydrocarbons, 102
hyperactivity, 96, 126-31
hypoglycaemia, 147-8, 149

ibuprofen, 110
IgA, 93, 115
IgE (Immunoglobulin E), 31, 77,
  84, 111
Illich, Ivan, Medical Nemesis, 163
immunity, 13; see also
  autoimmunity
Immunoglobulin E, see IgE
immunology, 28-32
indigestion, 37
individual feeding test, 177
indomethacin, 110
infants: and allergies, 114-21
influenza, 29, 137
insecticides, 59, 64
Intal, 112
itching, 96

Jackson, Dr Alan, 115-17
Journal of Allergy, 42-3
Journal of Immunology, 38

Kaiser Permanente Medical
  Center, San Francisco, 129
Kansas City, 34
Kay, S.R., 140
King's College Hospital,
  London, 57
King, David, 77-8
Klee, W.A., 141-2
Kosterlitz, Hans, 141
Kustner, Heinz, 27
Kwok, Robert, 57, 65

Lachance, P.A., 66
lactase, 71, 115-16
lactose, 65, 71, 116
lamb, 10, 99, 134
Lancet (journal), 20, 33-4,
  115-17, 136, 144
Lawson, Ray, 150
lead poisoning, 127-8
lead pollution, atmospheric,
  127
leather, 103
lecithin, 65
Lee, Carlton, 75-6, 79
Lee, Mrs Carlton, 75
livetin, 65
Lockey, Stephen, 56
Lodge-Rees, E., 127
LSD, 101
Lucretius, 13

Mackarness, Richard, 24-5, 38,

118, 147, 150; Not All in the
  Mind, 137
MacNulty, Alan, 21-2
macrobiotics, 165
Manchester, 26
Mandell, Marshall, 77-8, 101
mania, 96
Mansfield, John, 134
marmalade, 100
masked allergies, 152
mass-produced foods, 61-4
mast cells, 31
Mayo Clinic, the, 15-16
McCarrison, Sir Robert, 166-8
McEwen, Leonard, 83-93, 96-7
  100, 147-8
McKeown, Thomas, The Role of
  Medicine: Dream, Mirage or
  Nemesis?, 163
measles, 29
meat extracts, 133
meat, 118; see also individual
  types
medicines, 62, 100, see also
  individual kinds
melatonin, 139
Ménière's syndrome, 34
mental disorders, 132-45; see
  also individual disorders
mercury, 128
Middlesex Hospital Medical
  School, London, 80
migraine, 33, 37, 71-3, 96-7,
  132-45, 151
milk, 15-16, 31, 34-5, 54, 65,
  70-71, 86, 89, 98, 100, 110,
  115-22, 135, 149, 159
Miller, Joseph, 79
monoamine oxidase, 133, 153
monosodium glutamate, 65
moonshine, 128
morphine, 139
moulds, 69, 101
mouthwash, 100
mushrooms, 135
mussels, 109-10

Nalcrom, 112
naloxone, 139, 148
National Health Institute (US),
  148
National Institute of Mental
  Health Research (US), 141
Nature (magazine), 63
New England Journal of Medicine,
  58
New York, 128
Nicholson, Norman, 58
nitrates, 58-9
nitrites, 58, 64
'Noon units', 80
Noon, L., 27, 80, 82
Northwestern University, 43-4
Nulacin, 125
numbness, 96
nuts, 31, 89, 100, 119

O'Shea, James, 130
Oakland, 35, 38
oats, 122
obesity, 14, 146-54
oil, 105
oil, olive, 99
onions, 89
oranges, 100, 119, 129, 135,
  159
osteoarthritis, see arthritis
ovocumin, 65
ovomucoid, 65
ovovitellin, 65
oxygen, 31

panic, attacks of, 96
peanuts, 159

pears, 99, 134
peas, 135
penicillin, 101
Pennington, Alfred, 150
Pennsylvania, University of,
  139
peptides, 141
Pepys, Jack, 69-70
period pains, 37
pesticides, 10, 63-5
pewter, 128
phenol, 102, 105
Philpott, William, 149
phosphates, 186
pica, 128
Pickering, Sir George, 172
pill, contraceptive, 12-13, 133-4
piperonyl butoxide, 63
Piriton, 57
placebos, 18-19, 77-9, 91
plastics, 102
platinum salts, 80
pneumonitis, 102
pollen, 26-7, 29-30, 79-80, 82,
  93, 100, 119
polyps, 97
Popper, Dr, 89-91
pork, 89, 100, 159
Porter, James, 130
potatoes, 100
Pottenger, Francis, 169-70
Potter, Robert, 22
Prausnitz, Carl, 27
preservatives, 64, 100, 184
prick tests, 80, 93
prostaglandins, 108-11, 139
protamine, 92-3
proteins, 29, 71, 115, 117
provocation tests, 78
pulse test, 177-8
pulse, racing, 96
Pure Food and Drug Act (USA,
  1906), 61
PVC, 103

raisins, 100
Randolph, Theron G., 10-11,
  43-54, 66-8, 102, 105, 147,
  150-53, 158-9
Rapp, Doris, 77; and A.W.
  Frankland, Allergies:
  Questions and Answers, 119
rashes, 96, 112-13, 128-9
Rea, Dr William, 105
Recent Advances in Allergy, 37
rheumatism, 155
rheumatoid arthritis, see
  arthritis
rhinitis, 83, 89, 96-7, 113
rice, 99
Richet, Dr, and Dr Saint Girons,
  L'Anaphylaxie Alimentaire, 35
Rinkel, Herbert, 40-43, 53,
  75-6, 97-8, 152
Ritalin, 126
Rowe, Albert, 35-8, 96
Royal College of Physicians
  (UK), 64
Royal College of Surgeons
  (UK), 90
Royal Society, the, 60
Rutgers University, 66
rye, 99, 122, 139-40
Rynacrom, 112

Saint Anthony's fire, 101
Saint Girons, Dr, see Richet, Dr,
  and Dr Saint Girons
salicylates, 100, 108, 129-30
salt, 65
Savage, George, 72
schizophrenia, 14, 71-3, 96,
  137-45
Schloss, Dr Oscar, 34

Schofield, Dr A.T., 34
Science (journal), 128, 140, 148
Scientific American (journal), 128
seafood, 171; see also fish;
    shellfish
Selye, Hans, 51-3
sequestrants, 187
shellfish, 31, 100, 110
Sikhs, 167-8
Silver, Francis, 103-4
Singh, M.M., 140
smoking, 12
sodium caseinate, 65
soft drinks, 100
solvents, 185-6
soreness, 96
South Africa, 156
spasms, 96
spores, 100
St Bartholomew's Hospital,
    London, 122
St Mary's Hospital, London,
    27, 55, 80-81, 91, 147
stabilizers, 184-5
starch, 33
steroids, synthetic, 112
stomach troubles, 97, 151; see

also individual conditions
'Stone Age Diet', 118, 150
strawberries, 35, 84, 100
streptomycin, 101
stress, 51-2, 134
Strong, Jim, 15-16
sublingual and intradermal
    'switch-on/switch-off', 93,
    99, 105, 178
Sugar Research Foundation, 67
sugar, 33, 65, 67-8 105, 118,
    135, 159
symptoms, 98; see also diagnosis

tanning chemicals, 103
tartrazine, 56, 100, 128-9
tea, 17-18, 135, 159
Temple University,
    Philadelphia, 148
tetanus, 29
thalidomide, 64
Thames Water Authority, the,
    58
Times, The (newspaper), 154
tobacco, 100; see also smoking
toluene di-isocyanate, 68
tomatoes, 48, 100, 111, 119,
    159

toothpaste, 100
Type Four allergy, 77, 175-6
Type One allergy, 30-31, 84, 89,
    173
Type Three allergy, 174-5
Type Two allergy, 173-4
tyramine, 97, 133

ulcerative colitis, 83
ulcers: aphthous, 22-3; gastric,
    37; duodenal, 37; mouth,
    37, 96; stomach, 14-16
United States of America, 28-9,
    37, 43, 59, 126, 128, 141
units, environmental, 105-6
urethane foam, 103
urticaria, 56

vaccination, 29; see also
    immunology
vegans, 163-5
vegetables, fresh, 118
vegetables, green, 99
vegetarians, 163-5
Ventolin, 57
vertigo, 96, 101
viruses, 29

vitamin C, 66
vitamins, 164-6, 170-71
vitellin, 65
vomiting, 96, 109
von Pirquet, Clemens, 13

Wagemaker, Dr, 143
Walker, Vera, 72-3
water melon, 35
Wattenburg, Lee, 171
weed killers, 64
wheat, 34-5, 59, 65, 89, 97-8,
    100, 122, 135, 139-40, 144,
    147, 159
whisky, 67-8; see also alcohol
Wiley, Harvey W., 61
wine, 57, 100, 110; see also
    alcohol; wine, red
wine, red, 97, 133
World Health Organization, 58,
    124
World Medicine (journal), 168-9

yeast, 65, 89, 133, 135
yogurt, 55

zinc, 127, 139